2016-2017
HESI Live Review Workbook for the
NCLEX-RN EXAM

ELSEVIER

ELSEVIER

3251 Riverport Lane
St. Louis, Missouri 63043

Library of Congress Cataloging-in-Publication Data

2016-2017 HESI live review workbook for the NCLEX-RN exam / Rosemary Pine, PhD, RN, BC, CDE, Director, Review Courses, Elsevier Review and Testing, Nursing and Health Professions, Houston, Texas [and five others] ; editors, Rosemary Pine, PhD, RN, BC, CDE, Director, Review Courses, Elsevier Review and Testing, Nursing and Health Professions, Houston, Texas, Ashley Mezger, MA, associate e-project manager, Elsevier Review and Testing, Nursing and Health Professions, Houston, Texas.
     pages cm
1. Practical nursing--Examinations, questions, etc. 2. Practical nursing--Outlines, syllabi, etc. I. Pine, Rosemary. II. Mezger, Ashley. III. Title: HESI live review workbook for the NCLEX-RN exam.
  RT55.H48 2016
  610.7306'93076--dc23

2015028597

Senior Content Strategist: Yvonne Alexopoulos
Content Development Manager: Laurie Gower
Senior Content Development Specialist: Lisa P. Newton
Publishing Services Manager: Hemamalini Rajendrababu
Project Manager: Maria Bernard
Designer: Xiaopei Chen/Ryan Cook

Printed in United States

Last digit is the print number: 9 8 7 6 5 4 3 2

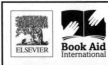

Contributors

Rosemary Pine, PhD, RN, BC
Director, Review Courses
Elsevier Review and Testing
Nursing and Health Professions
Houston, TX

E. Tina Cuellar, PhD, RN
Director, Curriculum
Elsevier Review and Testing
Nursing and Health Professions
Houston, TX

Julia Vicente, MSN, RN, CCRN-K
Adjunct Professor
Chamberlain College of Nursing
Miramar, FL

Marcia L. Gasper, EdD, RN
Associate Professor of Nursing
East Stroudsburg University
East Stroudsburg, PA

Helen Freeman, MSN, RN-BC, CNE
Consultant
Mars Hill, NC

Virginia J. Hallenbeck, DNP, RN, ACNS-BC
Clinical Nurse Specialist/Adjunct Faculty
Ohio State University Medical Center
Columbus, OH

Diane E. Friend, MS, RN, CDONA/LTC
Assistant Professor
Allegany College of Maryland
Cumberland, MD

Barbara Magenheim, EdD, RN, CNE
Nursing Faculty
Chandler Gilbert CC
Mesa, AZ

Holly J. Diesel, PhD, RN
Associate Professor
Goldfarb School of Nursing at Barnes-Jewish College
St. Louis, MO

Lisa Kritz, MA, RNC-OB
Clinical Specialist
Mercy Medical Center
Dubuque, IA

Amber Essman, DNP, APRN, FNP-BC, CNE
Professor
Indiana University East
Richmond, IN

JoAnne Gaudet, MSN, RN, CCRN
Clinical Educator
Houston Methodist Hospital
Houston, TX

*The editors and publisher would like to acknowledge the
following individuals for contributions to the previous editions of the book.*

Susan Morrison, PhD, RN
President Emerita
Elsevier Review and Testing
Nursing and Health Professions
Houston, TX

Ainslie Nibert, PhD, RN, FAAN
Associate Dean
Nursing and Health Professions
Texas Woman's University
Houston, TX

Mickie Hinds, PhD, RN
Former Director, Review and Curriculum
Elsevier Review and Testing
Nursing and Health Professions
Houston, TX

Judy Siefert, MSN, RN
Director, Testing
Elsevier Review and Testing
Nursing and Health Professions
Houston, TX

Denise Voyles, MS, RN
Testing Manager
Elsevier Review and Testing
Nursing and Health Professions
Houston, TX

Sandra L. Upchurch, PhD, RN
Former Director, Curriculum
Elsevier Review and Testing
Nursing and Health Professions
Houston, TX

Traci Henry, MSN, RN
Former Curriculum Manager
Elsevier Review and Testing
Nursing and Health Professions
Houston, TX

Marilyn Tompkins, DrPH, RN, FNP, BC
Family Nurse Practitioner
Lakeside-Milam Recovery Centers
Kirkland, Washington

Cathy Griteman, MSN, RN
Testing Manager
Elsevier Review and Testing
Nursing and Health Professions
Houston, TX

1 Test-Taking Strategies and Study Guide

Welcome to the HESI Live Review Course

This series of slides and the workbook provide test-taking strategies, sample test questions, and a content review of the nursing curriculum to help prepare nursing students for the NCLEX-RN examination. For a more in-depth review of certain material, please refer to the following:

- *HESI Comprehensive Review for the NCLEX-RN Examination*
- *Mosby's Comprehensive Review of Nursing for the NCLEX-RN Examination*
- *HESI/Saunders Online Review for the NCLEX-RN Examination*

Knowledge is power!

Goals of the Live Review Course

- Strengthen test-taking skills
  - Incorporate recommended strategies to manage anxiety
  - Formulate a study plan using tools such as the *HESI Live Review Workbook for the NCLEX-RN Exam*
- Review basic curriculum content

NLCEX-RN Examination

About the NCLEX-RN Blueprint

- The tests cover essential nursing knowledge.
- The test plan is revised every 3 years after a practice analysis has been conducted with entry-level nurses.
- Information about the test plan, including descriptions of content categories and related content for each category, can be found on the website for the National Council of State Boards of Nursing (www.ncsbn.org).
- The NCSBN website also presents information for students, frequently asked questions, and examples of alternate formats.
- The content of the NCLEX-RN Test Plan is organized into four major client needs categories. Two of the four categories are divided into subcategories:
  - Safe and Effective Care Environment
    - Management of Care
    - Safety and Infection Control
  - Health Promotion and Maintenance
  - Psychosocial Integrity
  - Physiological Integrity
    - Basic Care and Comfort
    - Pharmacological and Parenteral Therapies
    - Reduction of Risk Potential
    - Physiological Adaptation

Processes

Processes fundamental to RN practice are integrated into all client needs categories.

- Nursing process
  - Planning and implementing nursing care based on assessment, diagnosis, and determining priorities
  - Evaluating the effectiveness of nursing care
- Caring
- Communication and documentation
- Teaching and learning

About Test Administration

With computerized adaptive testing (CAT), the difficulty of the exam is tailored to the candidate's ability level. All RN candidates must answer a minimum of 75 items. The maximum number of items the candidate may answer during the allotted 6-hour period is 265.

About Test Item Questions

Multiple-choice items
- Comprise the majority of items
- One question with four choices (answers) from which to choose the correct response

Multiple-response items
- Require the candidate to select one or more than one response from five to seven choices
- The candidate is instructed to select all that apply

Fill-in-the-blank items
- Require a candidate to type in one or more numbers in a calculation item
- If rounding is necessary, it is performed at the end of the calculation

Hot spot items
- Instruct the candidate to identify one or more areas on a picture or graphic
- Can measure skills related to safety, physical assessment, and other procedures and techniques

Chart/exhibit format
- Presents the candidate with a problem that requires the individual to read the information in the chart/exhibit to arrive at the answer
- Provides the client history, laboratory data, and clinical data on tabs

Ordered response items or drag and drop
- Require a candidate to rank order or move options to provide the correct answer
- Presents the candidate with a list of the essential steps of a nursing procedure (e.g., cardiopulmonary resuscitation—CPR) and instructs the individual to order the steps in the correct sequence

Audio item format
- Presents the candidate with an audio clip; the individual uses headphones to listen to the question and select the answer option that applies
- Evaluates the candidate's competence in certain skills or assessment areas

Graphic options
- May be used as all or part of an individual item, either in the question itself or as part of the response

Test-Taking Strategies

General Strategies
- Every question must be answered to move to the next question, so make your best guess if you are not sure of the answer.
- Quickly eliminate the options that do not answer the question.
- Reread the question for qualifiers or other words that specify what the question asks.
- Decide what makes the responses different from each other.
- Keep in mind that the choice may contain correct information but may not answer the question.

For Your Toolbox
- Use the *ABCs* when selecting an answer or determining the order of priority.
  — Remember the order of priority: airway, breathing, and circulation.
  — The exception to the rule, which is with actual CPR, is C-A-B.
- Maslow's Hierarchy of Needs
  — Address physiological needs first, followed by safety and security needs, love and belonging needs, self-esteem needs, and finally self-actualization needs.
  — When a physiological need is not addressed in the question, look for the option that addresses safety.
- Carefully read the question to determine the step of the nursing process.
  — *Assessment* questions address the gathering and verification of data.
  — *Analysis* questions require the nurse to:
    - Interpret data and collect additional information
    - Identify and communicate nursing diagnoses
    - Determine the health team's ability to meet the client's needs
- *Planning* questions ask about determining, prioritizing, and modifying outcomes of care.
- *Implementation* questions reflect the management and organization of care and the assignment and delegation of tasks. Be prepared for questions on client teaching.
- *Evaluation* questions focus on comparing the actual outcomes of care with the expected outcomes and on communicating and documenting findings.

- Think: safety, safety, SAFETY!
- Start with the least invasive intervention.
- Assess before taking action, when appropriate.
- Have all necessary information and take all possible relevant actions before calling the physician/health-care provider.
- Determine which client to assess first (i.e., most at risk, most physiologically unstable).
- Follow guidelines for delegating assignments.
- Remember the differences between the role of the licensed nurse and the role of unlicensed assistive personnel (UAP).

The Question May Contain "Red Flag" Words

Practice rewording the following questions:
1. "Which response indicates to the nurse a need to re-teach the client about …."
2. "Which prescription (order) should the nurse question?"

Common Interventions

- Small, frequent feedings
- Recommended fluid intake: "3 L/day"
- Alternate rest with activity
- Conserve energy with any activity

Teaching Points

- Risk factors—known modifiable versus nonmodifiable
- Prevention and wellness promotion
- New medications/self-care instructions
- Client empowerment
- Anticipatory guidance
- Incorporating client education information into the client's lifestyle, culture, spiritual beliefs, and so on

A Few Words About "Words"

Health care provider (HCP): The person prescribing care (e.g., physician, nurse practitioner)
Prescriptions: Orders written by licensed health care providers
Unlicensed assistive personnel (UAP)
- Client care technician
- Nursing assistant
- Nurse's aide

Keep Memorizing to a Minimum

- Growth and developmental milestones
- Death and dying stages
- Crisis intervention
- Immunizations
- Drug classifications
- Principles of teaching/learning
- Stages of pregnancy and fetal growth
- Nurse Practice Act: Standards of Practice and Delegation

Practice Rewording

1. _____
2. _____

Strategies for Success in Answering NCLEX-RN Questions: Four Essential Steps

1. Determine whether the style of the question is

\+ positive +

or

− negative −

2. Find the key words in the question.
3. Rephrase the question in your own words and then answer the question.
4. Rule out options.

Determine Whether the Question Is Written in a Positive or Negative Style

- A *positive style* may ask what the nurse should do or the best or first action to implement.
- A *negative style* may ask what the nurse should avoid, which prescription the nurse should question, or which behavior indicates the need for reteaching the client.

Find the Key Words in the Question

- Ask yourself which words or phrases provide the critical information.
- This information may be the age of the client, the setting, the timing, a set of symptoms or behaviors, or any number of other factors.
- For example, the nursing actions for a 10-year-old, 1-day postoperative client are different from those for a 70-year-old, 1-hour postoperative client.

Rephrase the Question in Your Own Words and Answer the Question

- This will help you to eliminate nonessential information in the question and to determine the correct answer.
- Ask yourself, "What is this instructor *really* asking?"
- Before looking at the choices, rephrase the question in your own words.
- Answer the question.

Rule Out Options

- Based on your knowledge, you can probably identify one or two options that are clearly incorrect.
- Mentally mark through those options on the computer monitor.
- Now differentiate among the remaining options, considering your knowledge of the subject and related nursing principles, such as the roles of the nurse, the nursing process, the ABCs, and Maslow's Hierarchy of Needs.

A hospitalized client reports to the nurse that he has not had a bowel movement in 2 days. Which intervention should the nurse implement first?

A. Instruct the caregiver to offer a glass of warm prune juice at mealtimes.
B. Notify the health care provider and request a prescription for a stool softener.
C. Assess the client's medical record to determine his normal bowel pattern.
D. Instruct the caregiver to increase the client's fluids to five 8-ounce glasses per day.

HESI Test Question Approach			
Positive?		YES	NO
Key Words			
Rephrase			
Rule Out Choices			
A	B	C	D

A client who has chronic obstructive pulmonary disease (COPD) is resting in a semi-Fowler's position with oxygen at 2 L/min per nasal cannula. The client develops dyspnea. What action should the RN take first?

A. Call the healthcare provider.
B. Obtain a bedside pulse oximeter.
C. Raise the head of the bed higher.
D. Assess the client's vital signs.

HESI Test Question Approach			
Positive?		YES	NO
Key Words			
Rephrase			
Rule Out Choices			
A	B	C	D

Specific Areas of Content

Laboratory Values

Know the normal ranges for commonly used laboratory tests, what variations mean, and the *best* nursing actions.

- Hemoglobin and hematocrit (H & H)
- White blood cells (WBCs), red blood cells (RBCs), platelets
- Electrolytes: K^+, Na^+, Ca^{2+}, Mg^{2+}, Cl^-, PO_4
- BUN and creatinine
- Relationship of Ca^{2+} and PO_4
- Arterial blood gases (ABGs)
- PT (prothrombin time), international normalized ratio (INR), partial thromboplastin time (PTT) (don't get them confused)

A client who has hyperparathyroidism is scheduled to receive a prescribed dose of oral phosphate. The RN notes that the client's serum calcium level is 12.5 mg/dL. What action should the nurse take?

A. Hold the phosphate and notify the healthcare provider.
B. Review the client's serum parathyroid hormone level.
C. Give an as-needed (PRN) dose of intravenous (IV) calcium per protocol.
D. Administer the dose of oral phosphate.

HESI Test Question Approach			
Positive?		YES	NO
Key Words			
Rephrase			
Rule Out Choices			
A	B	C	D

In completing a client's preoperative routine, the RN finds that the operative permit has not been signed. The client begins to ask more questions about the surgical procedure. What action should the nurse take next?

A. Witness the client's signature on the permit.
B. Answer the client's questions about the surgery.
C. Inform the healthcare provider that the client has questions about the surgery.
D. Reassure the client that the surgeon will answer any questions before the anesthetic is administered.

HESI Test Question Approach			
Positive?		**YES**	**NO**
Key Words			
Rephrase			
Rule Out Choices			
A	**B**	**C**	**D**

Nutrition

Be able to identify foods relative to their sodium content (high or low), potassium level (high or low), and increased levels of phosphate, iron, or vitamin K.

■ Chemotherapy, gastrointestinal/gastrourinary disturbances
■ Proteins, carbohydrates, fats
■ Pregnancy and fetal growth needs
■ Remember these concepts:
    — Introducing one food at a time (infants, allergies)
    — Progression "AS TOLERATED"
■ The nursing assessment that guides decisions about progression

Medication Administration and Pharmacology

Pharmacological treatment and related nursing implications are reviewed in each chapter to coincide with the disease processes and conditions of the client.

More critical thinking questions are being designed around SKILLS!

Think: safety, *safety,* SAFETY!

Reflect on … the *whole picture.*

Safe medication administration is more than just knowing the action of the medications. It also includes:

■ The "6 Rights" (six *plus* technique of skill execution)
    1. Right drug
    2. Right dose
    3. Right route
    4. Right time
    5. Right patient
    6. Right documentation
■ Drug interactions
■ Vulnerable organs (√ labs; what to assess)
■ Allergies and presence of suprainfections
■ Concept of peak and trough

How you would know:
■ Whether the drug is working
■ A problem has arisen

Teaching: *safety, empowerment, compliance*

Special Considerations

- Teratogens
- Vesicants
- Implications of edema, impaired tissue perfusion at injection site
- Relationship of hepatorenal status to drug dose/frequency
- Concepts of weaning

Practical Tips

When answering an NCLEX question:

Do not respond based on:

- *Your* past client care experiences or agency
- A familiar phrase or term
- "Of course, *I* would have already ..."
- What *you* think is *realistic*
- *Your* children, pregnancies, parents, elders, personal response to a drug, and so on

Do respond based on:

- ABCs
- Scientific, behavioral, sociological principles
- Principles of teaching/learning
- Maslow's Hierarchy of Needs
- Nursing process
- Answer based only on what the question asks—no more, no less
- NCLEX-RN ideal hospital
- Basic anatomy and physiology
- Critical thinking

Best Practice for a Successful NCLEX-RN Exam

Manage Anxiety Between Now and the Test

- Think positively and believe in yourself.
- Use positive self-talk ("I can do this!").
- Set up a study schedule and stick to it.
- Avoid negative people.
- Respect your body and your mind.
- Establish a balanced lifestyle (i.e., a regular schedule for sleeping, eating, exercising, socializing, and working).

Develop a Study Schedule

- Organize resources.
  - Online texts, hard copy books, review questions
  - Practice tests, case studies
- Identify your challenges; review these:
  - Results of your HESI Exit Exam
  - Final grades
  - Feedback on clinical performance
  - Results of practice tests
- Initially take practice tests specific to your areas of weakness.
- Establish a study schedule that includes adequate time to prepare.

- Know your testing date.
  — Plan your schedule for the 4 to 8 weeks before your testing date.
- Would a study group help you?
- Make sure you have a comfortable level of memorization of growth and development markers, lab results, drug categories, drug calculations, and immunization schedules.

A Week Before the Exam
- Take a test drive to the site.
- Be mindful of traffic patterns.
- Familiarize yourself with the test center.
- Confirm that you have all the documents you need to be admitted to the exam.

The Day Before the Test
- Allow only 30 minutes to review test-taking strategies.
- If you feel the need to, review your notes the night before the exam, but allow for a restful 7 to 8 hours of sleep.
- Assemble all necessary materials:
  — Admission ticket
  — Directions to testing center
  — Identification
  — Money for lunch
- Do something you enjoy.
- Respect your body and your mind.

The Day of the Test
- Eat a healthy meal.
- Allow plenty of time to get to the testing center.
- Dress comfortably.
- Take only your identification forms into the testing room.
- Avoid distractions.
- Use positive self-talk.

At the Exam
- Breathe deeply and regularly.
- Continue the positive self-talk.
- Be in the moment and take the exam; no regrets.
- Do not allow the number of questions to influence your level of self-confidence.

You can do this!

2 Legal Aspects and Clinical Management of Care

Legal Aspects

Legal Systems

- Civil law is concerned with the protection of the client's private rights.
- Criminal law deals with the rights of individuals and society as defined by legislative laws.

Nursing negligence is the failure to exercise the proper degree of care required by the circumstances that a reasonably prudent person would exercise under the circumstances to avoid harming others. It is a careless act of omission or commission that results in injury to another.

Nursing malpractice, often referred to as *professional negligence,* is a type of negligence. It is the failure to use that degree of care that a reasonable nurse would use under the same or similar circumstances.

Malpractice is found when:

- The nurse owed a duty to the client.
- The nurse did not carry out that duty or breached that duty.
- The client was injured.
- The nurse's failure to carry out that duty caused the client's injury.

Standards of Care

- Nurses are required to follow standards of care, which originate in Nurse Practice Acts, state and federal law (United States) and provincial, territorial, and federal laws (Canada), accreditation recommendations, the guidelines of professional organizations, and the written policies and procedures of the healthcare agency.
- Nurses are responsible for performing procedures correctly and exercising professional judgment when implementing healthcare providers' prescriptions.

The unlicensed assistive personnel (UAP) reports to a staff nurse that a client who had surgery 4 hours ago has had a decrease in blood pressure (BP), from 150/80 to 110/70, in the past hour. The nurse advises the UAP to check the client's dressing for excess drainage and report the findings to the nurse. Which factor is most important to consider when assessing the legal ramifications of this situation?

A. The parameters of the state's or province's nurse practice act.

B. The need to complete an adverse occurrence report.

C. Hospital protocols regarding the frequency of vital sign assessment every hour postoperatively.

D. The healthcare provider's prescription for changing the postoperative dressing.

HESI Test Question Approach			
Positive?		YES	NO
Key Words			
Rephrase			
Rule Out Choices			
A	B	C	D

In the elevator, the UAP overhears two nurses talking about a client who will lose her leg because of the negligence of the staff. What federal law has been violated?

A. Health Insurance Portability and Accountability Act (HIPAA)
B. Americans with Disabilities Act (ADA)
C. Nurse Practice Act (NPA)
D. Patient Self-Determination Act (PSDA)

HESI Test Question Approach			
Positive?		**YES**	**NO**
Key Words			
Rephrase			
Rule Out Choices			
A	**B**	**C**	**D**

Practice Issues

- Nurses must follow the healthcare provider's prescription unless the nurse believes that it is in error, that it violates hospital policy, or that it is harmful to the client.
- The nurse makes a formal report explaining the refusal.
- The nurse should file an incident (occurrence) report for any situation that may result in harm to the client.

Advance Directives (ADs)

- Assess the client's knowledge of advance directives.
- Integrate them into the client's plan of care.
- Provide the client with information about advance directives or review ADs on admission.
- Advance directives can limit life-prolonging measures when there is little or no chance of recovery.
- Living will: a client documents his or her wishes regarding future care in the event of terminal illness.
- Durable power of attorney for healthcare: a client appoints a representative (healthcare proxy) to make healthcare decisions.
  — The client must receive AD information or review ADs on admission.
  — Living wills and advance directives (Canada)
    • Instructional advance directives: gives directions on the level of health interventions
    • Proxy directive: names a substitute decision maker
    • Advance directives are evolving and vary throughout the provinces and territories.

An awake and alert client with impending pulmonary edema is brought to the emergency department. The client provides the nurse with a copy of a living will stating that "no invasive" medical procedures should be used to "keep her alive." The healthcare team is questioning whether the client should be intubated. What information should guide the team's decision?

A. The living will removes the obligation to involve the client in any medical decision making.
B. The client is awake and alert, which makes the living will irrelevant and nonbinding.
C. Lifesaving measures do not need to be explained to the client because of the signed living will.
D. The family should be contacted to determine who has durable power of attorney for healthcare for the client.

HESI Test Question Approach			
Positive?		**YES**	**NO**
Key Words			
Rephrase			
Rule Out Choices			
A	**B**	**C**	**D**

Restraints/Safety Reminder Devices (SRDs)

- Restraints and SRDs can be used *only:*
  - To ensure the physical safety of the client or other residents
  - When less restrictive interventions are not successful
  - On the written order of a healthcare provider
- The nurse must follow agency policy and procedure to restrain any client.
- Documentation of the use of restraints and of follow-up assessments must detail the attempts to use less restrictive interventions.
- Liability for improper or unlawful restraint lies with the nurse and the healthcare facility.

A family member of a client who is in a Posey vest restraint (safety reminder device) asks why the restraint was applied. How should the nurse respond?

A. The restraint was prescribed by the healthcare provider.

B. There are not enough staff members to keep the client safe all the time.

C. The other clients are upset when the client wanders at night.

D. The client's actions place her at high risk for harming herself.

HESI Test Question Approach			
Positive?		**YES**	**NO**
Key Words			
Rephrase			
Rule Out Choices			
A	B	C	D

Legal Aspects of Mental Health

- Admissions
  - Involuntary
  - Emergency
- Client's rights
- Competency

What nursing action has the highest priority when admitting a client to a psychiatric unit on an involuntary basis?

A. Reassure the client that the admission is only for a limited time.

B. Offer the client and family the opportunity to share their feelings about the admission.

C. Determine the behaviors that resulted in the need for admission.

D. Advise the client about the legal rights of all hospitalized clients.

HESI Test Question Approach			
Positive?		**YES**	**NO**
Key Words			
Rephrase			
Rule Out Choices			
A	B	C	D

Confidential Healthcare

- The Health Insurance Portability and Accountability Act of 1996 (HIPAA) established standards for the verbal, written, and electronic exchange of private health information.
- HIPAA created clients' rights to consent to use and disclose health information, to inspect and copy one's medical record, and to amend mistaken or incomplete information.
- HIPAA requires all hospitals and health agencies to have specific policies and procedures in place to ensure compliance with its standards.

The Personal Information Protection and Electronic Documents Act (PIPEDA) (Canada) is federal legislation that protects personal information, including health information. PIPEDA delineates how private-sector organizations may collect, use, or disclose personal information.

Informed Consent

Informed consent must meet the following criteria:

- The client giving consent is competent and of legal age.
- The consent is given voluntarily.
  - The client giving consent understands the procedure, its risks and benefits, and alternative procedures.
- The client giving consent has the right to have all questions answered satisfactorily.
- It is the duty of the healthcare provider who is performing the procedure or treatment to obtain informed consent.
- The RN is witnessing the signature, not providing informed consent.
- Answers to any questions the client has about a procedure are the responsibility of the healthcare provider who will perform the procedure.

The nurse enters the room of a preoperative client to obtain the client's signature on the surgical consent form. Which question is most important for the nurse to ask the client?

A. "When did the surgeon explain the procedure to you?"
B. "Is any member of your family going to be here during your surgery?"
C. "Have you been instructed in postoperative activities and restrictions?"
D. "Have you received any preoperative pain medication?"

Good Samaritan Laws

- Good Samaritan laws limit liability if a nurse offers assistance at the scene of an accident, as long as the nurse acts within acceptable standards of care.
- The nurse should provide only care that is consistent with his or her level of expertise.

HESI Test Question Approach			
Positive?		YES	NO
Key Words			
Rephrase			
Rule Out Choices			
A	B	C	D

Abuse

- The nurse has legal responsibilities related to reporting incidences of abuse, neglect, or violence.
- Healthcare professionals who do not report suspected abuse or neglect are liable for civil or criminal legal action.

Which assignment should the nurse delegate to a UAP in an acute care setting?
A. Hourly blood glucose checks for a client with a continuous insulin drip
B. Giving PO (by mouth) medications left at the bedside for the client to take after eating
C. Taking vital signs for an older client with left humeral and left tibial fractures
D. Replacing a client's pressure ulcer dressing that has been soiled by incontinence

HESI Test Question Approach		
Positive?	**YES**	**NO**
Key Words		
Rephrase		
Rule Out Choices		
A	B	C	D

Clinical Management of Care

Communication Skills

Types of leadership:
- "Do it my way."
  — Aggressive communication/authoritarian leader
- "Whatever . . . as long as you like me."
  — Passive communication/laissez-faire leader
- "Let's consider the options available."
  — Assertive communication/democratic leader

The charge nurse confronts a staff nurse whose behavior has been resentful and negative since a change in unit policy was announced. The staff nurse states, "Don't blame me; nobody likes this idea." What is the charge nurse's priority action?
A. Confront the other staff members involved in the change of unit policy.
B. Call a unit meeting to review the reasons the change was made.
C. Develop a written unit policy for the expression of complaints.
D. Encourage the nurse to be accountable for her own behavior.

HESI Test Question Approach		
Positive?	**YES**	**NO**
Key Words		
Rephrase		
Rule Out Choices		
A	B	C	D

Delegation Skills

Delegation is the process through which responsibility and authority—but *not* accountability—are transferred to another individual.
- The nursing process or any activity requiring nursing judgment may not be delegated to the UAP (unregulated care provider [UCP]).
- Five rights of delegation
  — Right task
  — Right circumstance

— Right person
— Right direction/communication
— Right supervision

The charge nurse is making assignments for each of four staff members, including a registered nurse (RN), a practical nurse (PN), and two UAPs (UCPs). Which task is best assigned to the PN?
A. Maintain a 24-hour urine collection.
B. Wean a client from a mechanical ventilator.
C. Perform sterile wound irrigation.
D. Obtain scheduled vital signs.

HESI Test Question Approach			
Positive?		**YES**	**NO**
Key Words			
Rephrase			
Rule Out Choices			
A	**B**	**C**	**D**

Supervision Skills

■ Direction/guidance
■ Evaluation/monitoring
■ Follow-up

Which situation warrants a variance (incident) report by the nurse?
A. A client refuses to take prescribed medication.
B. A client's status improves before completion of the course of medication.
C. A client has an allergic reaction to a prescribed medication.
D. A client received medication prescribed for another client.

HESI Test Question Approach			
Positive?		**YES**	**NO**
Key Words			
Rephrase			
Rule Out Choices			
A	**B**	**C**	**D**

Handoff Communication

■ A communication in which important client information is shared at pertinent points of care (e.g., change of shift, transfer from one clinical setting to another)
■ Ensures continuity of care and client safety
■ Improves communication and appropriate delegation

A nurse is preparing for change of shift. Which action by the nurse is characteristic of ineffective handoff communication?

A. The nurse states to the nurse coming on duty: "The client is anxious about his pain after surgery. Review the information I gave him about how to use an incentive spirometer."

B. The nurse refers to the electronic medical record (EMR) to review the client's medication administration record.

C. During rounds the nurse talks about the problem the UAP created by not performing a fingerstick blood glucose test on the client.

D. Before giving report, the nurse performs rounds on her assigned clients so that there is less likelihood of interruption during handoff.

S-BAR

S-BAR is an interdisciplinary communication strategy that promotes effective communication among caregivers.

S SITUATION—State the issue or problem.

B BACKGROUND—Provide the client's history.

A ASSESSMENT—Give the most recent vital signs and current findings.

R RECOMMENDATION—State what should be done.

The charge nurse is planning client assignments for the shift. The care team includes a registered nurse (RN), a practical nurse (PN), and unlicensed assistive personnel (UAP) on the care team. Which client(s) could be assigned to the PN? (Select all that apply.)

A. A client scheduled for a STAT x-ray after a fall on his hip

B. A client receiving IV vancomycin (Vancocin) through a peripherally inserted central catheter (PICC) line.

C. A client with sickle cell crisis who was transferred from the intensive care unit to the acute care area and who is receiving hydromorphone (Dilaudid) via a patient-controlled analgesia pump.

D. A client with a pressure ulcer who was prescribed negative pressure (wound VAC) care.

E. A postoperative client who has been prescribed two units of packed red blood cells.

A charge nurse is making assignments for five clients. The nursing team has an RN, a PN, and two UAPs. Which client(s) would be assigned to the RN? (Select all that apply.)

A. A client from the previous shift with unstable angina.

B. A client with a stage 3 pressure ulcer who needs a bed bath.

C. A client with an enteral feeding absorbing at 30 mL/hr.

D. A cardiotomy client who is day 2 postoperative and who has chest tubes.

E. A client with quadriplegia for whom urinary catheterization has been prescribed.

HESI Test Question Approach			
Positive?		YES	NO
Key Words			
Rephrase			
Rule Out Choices			
A	B	C	D

HESI Test Question Approach				
Positive?			YES	NO
Key Words				
Rephrase				
Rule Out Choices				
A	B	C	D	E

HESI Test Question Approach				
Positive?			YES	NO
Key Words				
Rephrase				
Rule Out Choices				
A	B	C	D	E

3 Clinical Concepts and Mechanisms of Disease

Perioperative Care

Perioperative is the broad tile and Preoperative is a subgroup under perioperative. See example below.

I. Perioperative care
  a. Preoperative
  b. Intraoperative
  c. Postoperative

Preoperative Care

- Preoperative evaluation
  — Obtain a complete history, including:
    • List of current medications (prescription, over the counter, complementary) and allergies
    • Previous surgical experiences (response to anesthetic)
    • Signed consent (confirm informed consent has been obtained before client is sedated)
- Preoperative teaching
  — Diet restrictions (typically NPO [nothing by mouth] after midnight before surgery)
  — Teach coughing and deep breathing, incentive spirometry
  — Review methods of pain control.

Intraoperative Care

- Maintain the client's safety.
- Surgical Care Improvement Project (SCIP) core measures are mandatory for client safety.
  — Emphasis is on preventing infection, serious cardiac events, and venous thromboembolism (VTE).
  — *Examples:* Administration of a prophylactic antibiotic within 1 hour of incision; glucose level <11.1 mmol/L (< 200 mg/dL); removal of urinary catheter on postoperative day 1 (POD #1) or POD #2; maintenance of beta-blocker therapy; provision of VTE prophylaxis
  — Mandatory time out
    • Confirm client's identity and consent, procedure to be performed, and surgical site.
- Provide psychosocial support.

Postoperative Care

- ABCs and hemodynamic stability (monitor for signs/symptoms of shock)
- Position client on side.
- Manage pain.

One of the primary goals of postoperative care is to prevent common complications.
- Urinary retention
  — Check for bladder distention.

- Urinary tract infection
  — Removal of urinary catheter POD #1 or POD #2
- Pulmonary problems
  — Check breath sounds.
  — Check O_2 saturation.
- Decreased peristalsis
- Paralytic ileus
- Absent bowel sounds
- Wound dehiscence
- Wound evisceration
- VTE

Pain

- Pain occurs in all clinical settings.
- Pain is whatever the client says it is.
- Pain is the fifth vital sign.
- Nurses have a central role in pain assessment and management.
- Assessment includes:
  — Subjective (P—Precipitating or palliative; Q—Quality or quantity; R—Region or radiation; S—Severity; T—Time)
  — Objective (pain rating scales and pain relief scales).
- Documentation includes: rating before and after medication, nonpharmacological measures initiated, patient teaching performed, and breakthrough pain measures implemented.
- The WHO (World Health Organization) recommends a stepwise approach to pain management.

Nonpharmacological Noninvasive Pain Relief Techniques

- Repositioning
- Heat and cold application
- Massage therapy
- Relaxation techniques
- Guided imagery
- TENS (transcutaneous electrical nerve stimulation)

Pharmacological Types of Pain Medications

- *Nonopioids* for mild pain or in combination for moderate pain
- *Opioids* for moderate to severe pain
- *Coanalgesic* or *adjuvant drugs* (i.e., anticonvulsants, antidepressants) for neuropathic pain

Nonopioid Analgesics
- Acetaminophen (Tylenol)
  — Maximum recommended dosage is 4,000 mg (4 g) in 24 hours.
  — Monitor liver and renal function.
  — Antidote: acetylcysteine
- Nonsteroidal anti-inflammatory drugs (NSAIDs) (nonselective)
  — Salicylates (Aspirin)
  — Ibuprofen (Motrin)
  — Ketorolac (Toradol)

— Indomethacin (Indocin)
— NSAIDs (selective)
- Cyclooxygenase-2 (COX-2) inhibitors
  — Celecoxib (Celebrex)

NSAIDs (except aspirin) have been linked to a higher risk for increased cardiovascular events, such as myocardial infarction, stroke, and heart failure. Clients who have just had heart surgery should not take NSAIDs.

Opioid Analgesics

- Mu agonists
  — Morphine sulfate (Dolorol, Kadian, M-Eslon, MS Contin)
  — Hydromorphone (Dilaudid)
  — Meperidine hydrochloride (Demerol, Pethidine)
  — Methadone hydrochloride (Methadol)
  — Levorphanol (Levo-Dromoran)
  — Fentanyl (Duragesic)
  — Oxycodone hydrochloride (Percocet, Percodan, Endocet, OxyContin, Oxy-IR, Supeudol)
  — Codeine sulfate
- Partial agonists
  — Buprenorphine hydrochloride
  — Butorphanol
  — Nalbuphine hydrochloride (Nubain)
  — Pentazocine hydrochloride (Talwin)
- Adjuvant drugs (used for neuropathic pain)
  — Anticonvulsants, antidepressants, and anesthetics are prescribed alone or in combination with opioids for neuropathic pain.
  — Corticosteroids

When opioids are prescribed for moderate pain, they are usually combined with a nonopioid analgesic, such as acetaminophen (e.g., codeine plus acetaminophen [Tylenol #3], hydrocodone plus acetaminophen [Vicodin]). Addition of acetaminophen or an NSAID limits the total daily dose that can be given.

Nonpharmacological Invasive Pain Relief Techniques

- Nerve blocks
- Interruption of neural pathways
- Spinal cord stimulation
- Acupuncture

A client has an order for hydromorphone (Dilaudid) intravenous (IV) push 1 mg every 3 hours. The drug is available as 4 mg/mL. The nurse administers _____ mL of hydromorphone for one dose. (Fill in the blank.)

Fluids and Electrolytes

Fluid Volume Excess

- Causes
  — Heart failure (most common), renal failure, cirrhosis, overhydration

- Symptoms
  - Peripheral edema, periorbital edema, elevated blood pressure, dyspnea, altered level of consciousness
- Lab findings
  - ↓ Blood urea nitrogen, ↓ hemoglobin, ↓ hematocrit, ↓ serum osmolality, ↓ urine specific gravity
- Treatment
  - Diuretics, fluid restrictions, weigh daily, monitor K^+

A client is transferred to the intensive care unit immediately after a craniotomy on a ventilator. IVs hanging are a fentanyl patient-controlled analgesia (PCA) pump, D5NS with 20 mEq KCl/L, and 1 unit of packed red blood cells with normal saline. The nurse reviews the medication administration record (MAR) and finds that the client reports an allergy to fentanyl and sulfamethoxazole-trimethoprim (cotrimoxazole). What action should the nurse take first?

A. Auscultate lung sounds for wheezing.
B. Notify the healthcare provider immediately.
C. Contact the healthcare proxy to verify allergies.
D. Stop the fentanyl PCA pump.

HESI Test Question Approach		
Positive?	YES	NO
Key Words		
Rephrase		
Rule Out Choices		
A	B	C	D

Fluid Volume Deficit
- Causes
  - Inadequate fluid intake
  - Hemorrhage
  - Vomiting, diarrhea
  - Massive edema
- Symptoms
  - Weight loss
  - Oliguria
  - Postural hypotension
- Laboratory findings
  - ↑ BUN
  - ↑ or normal creatinine (↑ Hgb, ↑ Hct, ↑ urine specific gravity)
- Treatment
  - Strict intake and output (I&O); replace with isotonic fluids
  - Monitor blood pressure
  - Weigh daily

Electrolyte Balance
- Intracellular (ICF)
  - K^+ maintains osmotic pressure.
  - K^+ imbalances may be life threatening.
- Extracellular (ECF)
  - Na^+ maintains most abundant osmotic pressure
  - Remember: When either the ECF or the ICF changes in concentration, fluid shifts from the area of lesser concentration to the area of greater concentration.

Types of Imbalances

Sodium (skeletal muscle contraction, cardiac contraction, nerve impulse transmission, and normal osmolarity and volume of the ECF)

Hyponatremia (diuretics, GI fluid loss, hypotonic IV fluids, diaphoresis)

- Na^+ <135 mmol/L (mEq/L)
- Muscle cramps, confusion, weakness, seizures
- Check blood pressure frequently.
- Restrict fluids, cautious IV saline replacement as needed

Hypernatremia (water deprivation, diabetes insipidus, renal failure, Cushing syndrome)

- Na^+ >145 mmol/L (mEq/L)
- Pulmonary edema, seizures, thirst, fever
- No IVs that contain sodium
- Restrict sodium in diet.
- Weigh daily

Potassium (depolarize and generate action potentials, regulating protein synthesis and glucose use and storage)

Hypokalemia (diuretics, vomiting, diarrhea, Cushing syndrome, gastric suction)

- K^+ <3.5 mmol/L (mEq/L)
- Rapid, thready pulse, flat T waves, fatigue, anorexia, muscle cramps
- IV potassium supplements
- Encourage foods high in K^+ (bananas, oranges, spinach).

Hyperkalemia (oliguria, acidosis, renal failure, Addison disease)

- K^+ >5.5 mmol/L (mEq/L)
- Tall, tented T waves, bradycardia, muscle weakness
- 10% to 20% glucose with regular insulin
- Kayexalate
- Renal dialysis

Calcium (maintaining bone strength and density, activating enzymes, allowing skeletal and cardiac muscle contraction, controlling nerve impulse transmission, and allowing blood clotting)

Hypocalcemia (renal failure, hypoparathyroidism, malabsorption, pancreatitis, alkalosis)

- Ca^{++} < 2.25 mmol/L (< 9.0 mEq/L)
- Positive Trousseau's sign, positive Chvostek's sign, diarrhea, numbness, convulsions
- Administer calcium supplements.
- IV calcium—give slowly
- Increase dietary calcium.

Hypercalcemia (hyperparathyroidism, malignant bone disease, excessive supplementation)

- Ca^{2+} >2.75 mmol/L (>10.5 mEq/L)
- Muscle weakness, constipation, nausea and vomiting, dysrhythmias, behavioral changes
- Limit vitamin D intake.
- Avoid calcium-based antacids.
- Administer calcitonin to reduce calcium.
- Renal dialysis may be required.

Magnesium (skeletal muscle contraction, carbohydrate metabolism, adenosine triphosphate [ATP] formation, vitamin activation, and cell growth)
Hypomagnesemia (alcoholism, malabsorption, diabetic ketoacidosis, diuretics)
■ Mg^{2+} <0.65 mmol/L (<1.3 mEq/L)
— Skeletal muscle weakness
— Hyperactive deep tendon reflexes
— Numbness and tingling
— Painful muscle contractions
— Decreased gastrointestinal (GI) motility, nausea

Hypermagnesemia (renal failure, adrenal insufficiency, excess replacement)
■ Mg^{2+} >1.05 mmol/L (>2.1 mEq/L)
— Bradycardia
— Peripheral vasodilation
— Hypotension
— Prolonged PR interval with a widened QRS complex
— Decreased to absent deep tendon reflexes

Phosphorus (activating vitamins and enzymes, forming ATP for energy supplies, assisting in cell growth and metabolism, maintaining acid-base balance and calcium homeostasis)
Hypophosphatemia (alcohol withdrawal, diabetic ketoacidosis, respiratory alkalosis)
■ Phosphate <.97 mmol/L (<3.0 mg/dL)
— Decreased cardiac output
— Weak peripheral pulses
— Skeletal muscle weakness

Hyperphosphatemia (renal failure, excess intake)
■ Phosphate >1.45 mmol/L (>4.5 mg/dL)
— Monitor for signs of hypocalcemia.

Which laboratory result for a preoperative client would prompt the nurse to contact the healthcare provider?
A. Platelet count: 151×10^9/L (151,000/mm^3)
B. White blood cell (WBC) count: 85×10^9/L (8500/mm^3)
C. Serum potassium level: 2.8 mmol/L (mEq/L)
D. Urine specific gravity: 1.031

HESI Test Question Approach			
Positive?		**YES**	**NO**
Key Words	.		
Rephrase			
Rule Out Choices			
A	B	C	D

IV Therapy
■ Types of IV fluids
— *Isotonic* (osmolarity between 270 and 300 mOsm/L): 0.9% normal saline (NS), LR (lactated Ringer's), D_5W (5% dextrose and water)
— *Hypotonic* (osmolarity less than 270 mOsm/L): 0.45% NS

— Hypertonic (osmolarity greater than 300 mOsm/L): D_5 0.45% NS, D_5LR, D5NS, D10W

▌Acid Base

The following are the basics for interpretation of arterial blood gas (ABG) results on the NCLEX-RN Exam.
- pH
  — Normal = 7.35 to 7.45
  — <7.35 = acidosis
  — >7.45 = alkalosis
- Pco_2
  — Normal = 35 to 45 mm Hg
  — >45 = acidosis
  — <35 = alkalosis
- Hco_3^-
  — Normal = 21 to 28 mmol/L (21 to 28 mEq/L)
  — <21 = acidosis
  — >28 = alkalosis

Arterial Blood Gas Interpretation Practice

Determine whether each set of ABGs indicates that the patient is normal, acidotic, or alkalotic. (Fill in the blank.)

1. pH = 7.32
   Pco_2 = 50
   Hco_3^- = 25
   This client is _____.

2. pH = 7.28
   Pco_2 = 35
   Hco_3^- = 18
   This client is _____.

3. pH = 7.43
   Pco_2 = 40
   Hco_3^- = 24
   This client is _____.

4. pH = 7.56
   Pco_2 = 44
   Hco_3^- = 38
   This client is _____.

5. pH = 7.33
   Pco_2 = 50
   Hco_3^- = 29
   This client is _____.

▌Safety

Sentinel Events
- An unexpected outcome involving a death or serious injury
- Signals the need for immediate investigation and response
- Accredited hospitals are expected to identify and respond to all sentinel events.
- Appropriate response includes:
  — Root cause analysis
  — Action plan designed to implement improvements to reduce risk
  — Implementation of improvements
  — Monitor the effectiveness of those improvements.

- Examples of sentinel events: patient suicide, operative/postoperative complication, wrong-site surgery, medication error, patient fall, patient death or injury in restraints, transfusion error

Falls
- Risk factors
  - *Adult:* Stroke, depression, mobility issues, history of seizure, history of falls, use of assistive devices, polypharmacy, environmental issues, forgetting or ignoring mobility issues
  - *Infants/children:* Length of stay, IV or saline lock, use of antiseizure medications, acute or chronic orthopedic diagnosis, receiving physical or occupational therapy, history of falls

Nursing and Collaborative Management
- Fall prevention
- Safety surveillance
- Assess need for pain relief, toileting, positioning
- Frequent reorientation
- Client and family education
- Address environmental concerns.
- Sitter

High-Alert Medications
- High-alert medications are most likely to cause significant harm to the client even when used as intended.
- Anticoagulants, narcotics and opiates, insulin, chemotherapeutic drugs, and sedatives are the most common high-alert medications.
- The most common types of harm associated with these medications are hypotension, bleeding, hypoglycemia, delirium, lethargy, and bradycardia.
- Strategies to prevent harm
- Built-in redundancies
- Double-checking
- Smart pumps
- Standardized or protocol order sets

A client is receiving an infusion of dobutamine hydrochloride. The order reads: Infuse dobutamine IV at 5 mcg/kg/min. 500 mg in 250 mL D5W. The client weighs 65 kg. Calculate the flow rate in mL/hr.
The flow rate is _____ mL/hr.

Death and Grief
- Stages of grief
  - Denial
  - Anger
  - Bargaining
  - Depression
  - Acceptance
- Encourage the client to express anger.
- Do not take away the defense mechanism or coping mechanism the client uses in a crisis.

- Customs surrounding death and dying vary among cultures.
- The nurse must make every attempt to understand and accommodate the family's cultural traditions when caring for a dying client.

Infection

- Invasion of the body by a pathogen
- Response to the invasion
- Localized
- Systemic
- Nosocomial infections
  — Acquired as a result of exposure to a microorganism in a hospital setting

Human Immunodeficiency Virus (HIV)
Routes of Transmission

- Unprotected sexual contact
  — Most common mode of transmission
- Exposure to blood through drug-using equipment
- Perinatal transmission
  — Most common route of infection for children
  — Can occur during pregnancy, at the time of delivery, or after birth through breastfeeding

Laboratory Testing

- Positive result on enzyme immunoassay (EIA) formally enzyme-linked immunosorbent assay (ELISA) and confirmed with Western blot test
- *A diagnosis of AIDS requires that the person be HIV positive and have either a CD4 + T-cell count of less than 200 cells/mm³ or an opportunistic infection*
- Polymerase chain reaction (PCR) (used with neonate)
- OraQuick In-Home HIV Test: Positive result is only preliminary; it must be confirmed by a healthcare professional

Nursing Assessment
Symptoms

- May begin with flulike symptoms in the earliest stage and advance to:
  — Fatigue, severe weight loss, swollen glands, unexplained fever, night sweats, dry cough
  — Secondary infections
  — Cancers
  — Neurological disease

Nursing and Collaborative Management

- Monitor stages of HIV disease progression and immune function (CD4 T-cell count).
- Initiate and monitor *highly active antiretroviral therapy (HAART)* (missing one dose might render the medications ineffective against the disease).
- Prevent development of opportunistic diseases (*Pneumocystis carinii* pneumonia [PCP], candidiasis, cytomegalovirus (CMV), tuberculosis).
- Detect and treat opportunistic diseases.

- Manage symptoms.
- Prevent or decrease complications of treatment.
- Prevent transmission of HIV.

Ongoing assessment, interaction with the client, and client education and support are required to accomplish these objectives.

HIV Drug Therapy

The goals of drug therapy are to:
- Reduce the viral load
- Maintain or raise the CD4+ T-cell counts
- Delay the development of HIV-related symptoms and opportunistic diseases

Nursing and Collaborative Management

- The client should have regular blood counts to track CD4 levels and the viral load.
- Side effects are common, and there are many drug-drug interactions.

HIV Medications

- Nucleoside reverse transcriptase inhibitors (NRTIs)
  — Zidovudine (AZT, Retrovir)
  — Didanosine (ddI, Videx)
  — Lamivudine (3TC, Epivir-HBV, Heptovir)
  — Abacavir sulfate (Ziagen)
  — Stavudine (d4T, Zerit)
  — Emtricitabine (Emtriva)
  — Tenofovir disoproxil (Viread)
- Non-nucleoside reverse transcriptase inhibitors (NNRTIs)
  — Nevirapine (Viramune)
  — Delavirdine mesylate (Rescriptor)
  — Efavirenz (Sustiva)
  — Protease inhibitors (PIs)
  — Indinavir sulfate (Crixivan)
  — Ritonavir (Norvir)
  — Nelfinavir mesylate (Viracept)
  — Atazanavir (Reyataz)
  — Fosamprenavir (Telzir)
- Fusion inhibitors
  — Enfuvirtide (Fuzeon)
- Entry inhibitor
  — Maraviroc (Selzentry)

Pediatric HIV

Common clinical manifestations of HIV infection in children include:
- Recurrent infections such as thrush
- Unexplained fever
- Lymphadenopathy
- Hepatosplenomegaly
- Oral candidiasis
- Failure to thrive
- Developmental delay

Considerations
- Client education concerns transmission and control of infectious diseases.
- Safety issues include appropriate storage of special medications and equipment.
- Prevention is a key component of HIV education.
- Aggressive pain management is essential.
- Common psychosocial concerns include disclosure of the diagnosis.
- Avoid exposure to individuals with infections (e.g., chickenpox).
- Administer no live viruses.
- If an HIV-infected mother is treated with zidovudine during pregnancy and the neonate is treated after birth, the probability of HIV infection of the child decreases from 30% to 4% to 8%.

Cancer

Chemotherapeutic Agents

Types of medications:
- Alkylating
  - Nitrogen mustards
  - Nitrosoureas
    - Antitumor antibiotic
    - Antimetabolite
    - Antimitotic (vinca alkaloids)
    - Topoisomerase inhibitors
    - Hormonal medications
    - Immunomodulator agents
    - Gene therapy
    - Targeted therapy
- Strict guidelines must be followed!
- These drugs normally are administered by a chemotherapy-certified nurse.
- Pregnant nurses should not administer most of these agents.
- Wear personal protective equipment for hazardous drug handling.
  - Gowns: disposable, made of fabric that has low-permeability to the agents in use, with closed-front and cuffs, intended for single use
  - Gloves: powder-free, labeled and tested for use with chemotherapy drugs, made of latex, nitrile, or neoprene.
  - Face and eye protection when splashing is possible
  - An approved respirator when there is a risk of inhaling drug aerosols (such as during spill or cleanup)
- Although the IV route is most common for administration, antineoplastic medication may be given by the oral, intra-arterial, isolated limb perfusion, or intra-cavitary route; dosing is usually based on the client's body surface area and type of cancer.
- Monitor for extravasation during infusion and notify the healthcare provider immediately if this occurs.
- Types of IV access devices used for administration:
  - Hickman
  - Broviac
  - Port-a-cath

- Side effects to monitor for after chemotherapy:
  — Mucositis
  — Alopecia
  — Anorexia, nausea, and vomiting
  — Diarrhea
  — Anemia
  — Low white blood cell count (neutropenia)
  — Thrombocytopenia
  — Infertility, sexual alterations

The complete blood count (CBC) results for a client receiving chemotherapy are: hemoglobin, 85 mmol/L (8.5 g/dL); hematocrit, 32%; WBC count, 6.5 × 109/L (6,500 cells/mm³). Which meal choice is best for this client?

A. Grilled chicken, rice, fresh fruit salad, milk
B. Broiled steak, whole wheat rolls, spinach salad, coffee
C. Smoked ham, mashed potatoes, applesauce, iced tea
D. Tuna noodle casserole, garden salad, lemonade

HESI Test Question Approach		
Positive?	YES	NO
Key Words		
Rephrase		
Rule Out Choices		
A	B	C	D

Care of the Client Receiving

Radiation Therapy

Types:
- External beam radiation (teletherapy)
- Brachytherapy

External beam (radiation source is external to the client)
- Instruct the client in self-care of the skin.
- Instruct not to remove the markings.

Brachytherapy (the radiation source comes into direct, continuous contact with the tumor tissue for a specific time; can include an unsealed source or sealed source)
- Client is *not* radioactive.
- Implants do contain radioactivity.
- Place client in private room.
- No pregnant caretakers or pregnant visitors
- Organize care to minimize exposure.
- Keep lead-lined container in room.
- All of client's secretions may be radioactive.
- Wear dosimeter film badge when providing care.
- Save bed linens and dressings until the source is removed, then dispose of in the usual manner.
- Other equipment can be removed from the room at any time.

Leukemia

- Risk factors: genetic, viral, immunological, and environmental factors, exposure to radiation, chemicals, and medications such as previous chemotherapy
- Types: lymphocytic and myelocytic or myelogenous
- Can be acute or chronic
- Affects the bone marrow causing anemia, leukopenia, thrombocytopenia, and immunosuppression

Classification of leukemia
- Acute lymphocytic leukemia (ALL)
  - Mostly lymphoblasts present in the bone marrow
  - Usually seen before 15 years of age
  - Favorable prognosis
- Acute myelogenous leukemia (AML)
  - Mostly myeloblasts present in the bone marrow
  - Onset between 15 and 39 years of age
  - Poor prognosis
- Chronic myelogenous leukemia (CML)
  - Mostly granulocytes in bone marrow
  - Age of onset is in the fourth decade
  - Poor prognosis
- Chronic lymphocytic leukemia (CLL)
  - Increased production of leukocytes and lymphocytes in the bone marrow, spleen, and liver
  - Clients usually 50 to 70 years of age
  - 5-year survival rate: 73% overall

Nursing Assessment

- Anorexia, fatigue, weakness, weight loss
- Fever, generalized lymphadenopathy, lethargy, epistaxis
- Integumentary: pallor or jaundice; petechiae, ecchymoses, purpura, reddish brown to purple cutaneous infiltrates, macules, and papules
- Cardiovascular: tachycardia, systolic murmurs
- Gastrointestinal: gingival bleeding and hyperplasia; oral ulcerations, herpes, and *Candida* infections; perirectal irritation and infection; hepatomegaly, splenomegaly
- Neurological: seizures, disorientation, confusion, decreased coordination, cranial nerve palsies, papilledema
- Musculoskeletal: muscle wasting, bone pain, joint pain
- Decreased hemoglobin and hematocrit, platelets; WBC count may be normal, elevated, or decreased depending on classification; positive bone marrow biopsy

Medications for Leukemia

- Chemotherapy
- Colony-stimulating factors
- Blood product replacement if indicated
- Administer IV antibiotics as ordered:
  - Trough (draw shortly before administration)
  - Peak (30 minutes to 1 hour after administration)

Nursing and Collaborative Management

- Monitor for infection, bleeding
- Report fever or signs/symptoms of infection to physician as soon as symptoms are recognized.
- Teach infection control measures.
- Provide high calorie, high protein, high carbohydrate diet.
- Ensure adequate rest and energy conservation.

Lymphomas

- Abnormal proliferation of lymphocytes
- Classifications depending on cell type
  - Hodgkin's (characterized by the presence of Reed-Sternberg cells in the nodes)
  - Non-Hodgkin's

- Risk factors
  — Viral infections, genetics
  — Sites of metastasis

The disease usually involves lymph nodes, tonsils, spleen, and bone marrow.

Nursing Assessment
- Enlarged lymph nodes, spleen, and liver
- Weight loss
- Fatigue
- Weakness
- Chills, fever, night sweats
- Tachycardia
- Anemia, thrombocytopenia
- Diagnostics
  — Positive biopsy of lymph nodes (cervical nodes affected first)
  — Presence of Reed-Sternberg cells in nodes
  — Positive computed tomography scan of liver and spleen

Nursing and Collaborative Management
- Stages I and II
  — External radiation and/or multiagent chemotherapy
  — Monitor for infection, bleeding, sterility—discuss the possibility for sperm banking with the male client

Multiple Myeloma
Abnormal number of plasma cells invades the bone marrow and destroy the bone with invasion of the lymph nodes, spleen, and liver
- Etiology: unknown
- Diagnostics
  — Presence of the Bence Jones protein in blood and urine
  — Increased levels of uric acid and calcium
  — Bone marrow aspiration positive for abnormal number of immature plasma cells

Nursing Assessment
- Pain (bone primarily in ribs, spine, and pelvis)
- Weakness, fatigue
- Anemia
- Osteoporosis
- Renal failure

Treatment
- Chemotherapy/external radiation
- Pain management
- Monitor for bone fractures, infection, bleeding, and signs of renal failure.
- Encourage at least 2 L of fluids per day.
- Blood products, antibiotics as indicated

A client is receiving vancomycin (Vancocin) IV and has a prescription for peak and trough levels. Before administering the next dose, what action should the nurse take?

A. Verify the culture and sensitivity results.
B. Review the client's WBC count.
C. Schedule the collection of blood for a peak level.
D. Determine whether the trough level has been collected.

HESI Test Question Approach			
Positive?		**YES**	**NO**
Key Words			
Rephrase			
Rule Out Choices			
A	**B**	**C**	**D**

Head and Neck Cancer

- Typically squamous cell in origin
- Tumor sites
- Paranasal sinuses
- Oral cavity
- Nasopharynx
- Oropharynx
- Larynx
- Significant disability because of the potential loss of voice, disfigurement, and social consequences
- Head and neck cancer is most common in men over age 50 and is related to heavy tobacco and alcohol intake.

Lung Cancer

- One of the leading causes of cancer-related deaths in Canada and the United States
- The increase in death rates for both men and women is directly related to cigarette smoking.
- Classified according to histological cell type
  — Small cell lung cancer (CSLC)
  — Non–small cell lung cancer (NSCLC)
  - Squamous cell
  - Adenocarcinoma
  - Large cell anaplastic
- Etiology/risk factors:
  — Cigarette smoking
  — Exposure to environmental and/or occupational pollutants

Nursing Assessment

- Symptoms of lung cancer are not usually apparent until the disease is in the advanced stages.
- Persistent hacking cough may be either dry or productive with blood-tinged sputum.
- Chest pain
- Hoarseness
- Dyspnea
- Abnormal chest radiograph
- Positive sputum on cytological examination

Treatment/Interventions

- Assess for tracheal deviation.
- Support oxygenation/ventilation.

- Diet: high calorie, high protein, high vitamin
- Nonsurgical
  — Chemotherapy
  — Radiation therapy
- Surgical intervention
  — Laser therapy
  — Thoracentesis
  — Thoracotomy with pneumonectomy—removal of entire lung
  — Thoracotomy with lobectomy—or segmental resection
- Nursing care depends on the type of medical treatment prescribed.

Postoperative Care

- Promote ventilation and re-expansion of the lung.
- Maintain a clear airway.
- Maintain the closed drainage system, if used.
- Promote arm exercises to maintain full use on the operative side.
- Promote good nutrition.
- Monitor incision for bleeding and subcutaneous emphysema.

Colorectal Cancer

Preventative screening:

At age 50: There is recommended preventative screening performed when one reaches the age of 50 for tests that screen for cancer.

- Test that primarily finds cancer
  — Stool for occult blood in the stool or fecal immunochemical test (FIT) yearly or stool DNA test every 3 years
- Tests that find polyps and cancer
  — Flexible sigmoidoscopy every 5 years*, or
  — Colonoscopy every 10 years, or
  — Double-contrast barium enema every 5 years*, or
  — Computed tomography colonography (virtual colonoscopy) every 5 years*
- The third most common form of cancer and the second leading cause of cancer-related deaths in the United States and Canada
  — Adenocarcinoma most common
  — Common metastasis to the liver
- Risk factors:
  — Age >50
  — Family history
  — History of chronic inflammatory bowel disease
  — History of ovarian or breast cancer

Nursing Assessment

- Blood in stool
- Change in bowel habits
- Abdominal pain, weight loss, nausea/vomiting
- Ribbonlike stool
- Sensation of incomplete evacuation

Treatment/Interventions
- Nonsurgical
- Pre- and/or postoperative radiation
- Postoperative chemotherapy

Surgical Intervention
- Bowel resection
- Temporary colostomy or ileostomy
- Permanent colostomy or ileostomy

Postoperative Care Issues
- Stoma care
- Incision care
- Abdominal
- Perineal
- Packing and drains
- HemoVac
- Jackson-Pratt

Stoma Assessment
- Stoma should be pink or red; ileostomy should be red
- Mild to moderate swelling of the stoma is normal for the first 2 to 3 weeks after surgery.
- Pouching system
- Skin barrier
- Bag or pouch
- Adhesive
- Help client cope with the stoma.
- Provide information.
- Teach practical stoma care techniques.
- Help client address issues involving social interactions.
- Employment
- Body image
- Sexuality

The nurse is caring for a client who is 24 hours post-procedure for a hemicolectomy with temporary colostomy placement. The nurse assesses the client's stoma, which is dry and dark blue. What action should the nurse take based on this finding?
A. Notify the healthcare provider of the finding.
B. Document the finding in the client's record.
C. Replace the pouch system over the stoma.
D. Place a petrolatum gauze dressing on the stoma.

HESI Test Question Approach			
Positive?		YES	NO
Key Words			
Rephrase			
Rule Out Choices			
A	B	C	D

Breast Cancer
- Preventative screening:
  - Monthly breast self-examination starting in their 20s
  - Recommend a mammogram yearly starting at the age 40 and continuing as long as a woman is in good health
  - Clinical breast examination about every 3 years for women in their 20s and 30s and every year for women 40 and over

- Common sites of metastasis: bone, lungs, brain, liver, and skin
- Risks
  — Family history
  — Age
  — Early menarche and late menopause
  — Obesity
  — Hyperestrogenism
  — Radiation exposure to chest

Nursing Assessment
- Mass: fixed, irregular, typically painless (usually felt in upper, outer quadrant, beneath the nipple, or in axilla)
- Nipple retraction or elevation
- Bloody or clear nipple discharge

Nursing and Collaborative Management
- Nonsurgical
- Chemotherapy
- Radiation therapy
- Hormonal manipulation (tamoxifen) for estrogen receptor positive tumors
- Biological-targeted therapies
- Monoclonal antibodies
- Surgical
- Lumpectomy
- Simple mastectomy
- Modified radical mastectomy with possible breast reconstruction
- Postoperative care
  — Monitor for bleeding, swelling, or fluid collection under the skin flaps on the arm.
  — Position arm on operative side on a pillow elevated above the level of the heart.
  — No blood pressure cuffs, IVs, or injections on operative side
  — Provide emotional support; recognize the grieving process; provide resources on support programs (e.g., Reach to Recovery).

Cancer of the Cervix
- Preventative screening:
  — Vaccinations against human papillomavirus (HPV)
  — Papanicolaou smear (Pap test)
- Cervical cancer screening (testing) should be within 3 years after having sexual intercourse or by the age of 21). Women between ages 21 and 29 should have a Pap test every 3 years; HPV testing should not be used in this age group unless it is needed after an abnormal Pap test result.
- Women between the ages of 30 and 65 should have a Pap test plus an HPV test (called "cotesting") every 5 years. This is the preferred approach, but it is also OK to have a Pap test alone every 3 years.
- Women over age 65 who have had regular cervical cancer testing with normal results should not be tested for cervical cancer; once testing is stopped, it should not be started again.

- Women with a history of a serious cervical precancer should continue to be tested for at least 20 years after that diagnosis, even if testing continues past age 65.
- A woman who has had her uterus removed (and also her cervix) for reasons not related to cervical cancer and who has no history of cervical cancer or serious precancer should not be tested.
- A woman who has been vaccinated against HPV should still follow the screening recommendations for her age group.
- Etiology: HPV infection, cigarette smoking, reproductive behaviors (first intercourse before 17, multiple partners)

Nursing Assessment
- Painless vaginal postmenstrual and postcoital bleeding
- Foul-smelling vaginal discharge
- Pelvic, lower back, leg, and/or groin pain
- Leakage of urine or stool from the vagina

Nursing and Collaborative Management
- Nonsurgical
  - Chemotherapy
  - Cryosurgery
  - External radiation
  - Internal radiation implants (intracavity)
- Surgical
  - Conization
  - Hysterectomy
  - Pelvic exenteration
- Postoperative care
  - Monitor bleeding (more than one saturated pad per hour may indicate excessive bleeding).
  - Monitor for infection.
  - Instruct client to avoid stair climbing for 1 month, tub baths, sitting for prolonged periods of time, strenuous activities, and heavy lifting (>20 pounds).

Ovarian Cancer
- Leading cause of death from gynecological cancer
- Greatest risk factor is family history
- Asymptomatic in early stages
- Generalized feeling of abdominal fullness
- Sense of pelvic heaviness
- Loss of appetite
- Change in bowel habits
- Late-stage symptoms
  - Pelvic discomfort
  - Low back pain
  - Abdominal pain

Testicular Cancer
- Preventative screening: monthly self-testicular examination
- Most often occurs between 15 and 40 years of age
- Etiology: unknown; history of cryptorchidism and genetic predisposition have been correlated with the development of the disease

Nursing Assessment

- Painless testicular swelling
- Feeling of heaviness in lower abdomen
- Palpable lymph nodes, abdominal masses, or gynecomastia may indicate metastasis; late signs include back or bone pain and/or respiratory symptoms

Nursing and Collaborative Management

- Encourage genetic counseling (sperm banking) before treatment
- Chemotherapy/radiation therapy
- Unilateral orchiectomy (for diagnosis or treatment or radical orchiectomy
- Postoperative
  — Observe for bleeding, infection
  — Pain management
  — Instruct the patient to avoid heavy lifting and strenuous activity; perform monthly testicular self-examination on the remaining testicle

Cancer of the Prostate

- Preventative screening
- Digital rectal exam (DRE)
- Prostate-specific antigen (PSA)
- Most prostate tumors are adenocarcinomas.
- Etiology/risk factors:
  — Advancing age
  — Heavy metal exposure
  — Smoking
  — History of sexually transmitted disease

Nursing Assessment

- Hard, pea-sized nodule palpated in rectal examination
- Gross, painless hematuria
- Symptoms of urinary obstruction
- Diagnostics: biopsy of the prostate gland

Nursing and Collaborative Management

- Nonsurgical
  — Hormone manipulation (leuprolide acetate, flutamide, or estrogens)
  — Radiation therapy (external beam or intracavitary)
  — Corticosteroids
  — Chemotherapy (in cases of hormone-resistant tumors)
- Surgical
  — Orchiectomy (palliative)
  — Transurethral resection of the prostate (palliative)
  — Prostatectomy cryosurgical ablation

The charge nurse is assigning rooms for four new clients. Only one private room is available on the oncology unit. Which client should be placed in the private room?

A. The client with ovarian cancer who is receiving chemotherapy.

B. The client with breast cancer who is receiving external beam radiation.

C. The client with prostate cancer who has just had a transurethral resection.

D. The client with cervical cancer who is receiving intracavitary radiation.

HESI Test Question Approach			
Positive?		YES	NO
Key Words			
Rephrase			
Rule Out Choices			
A	B	C	D

Brain Tumor

■ Primary malignant tumors can arise in any area of brain tissue.

■ Benign tumors can continue to grow and cause problems with ↑ intracranial pressure (ICP).

■ Nursing assessment

■ Assess for headache, vomiting, seizures, aphasia, and abnormal findings on computed tomography, magnetic resonance imaging, or positron emission tomography scan.

Nursing and Collaborative Management

■ Management is similar to that of a client with a head injury.

■ Major concern is ↑ ICP.

■ Keep head of bed elevated 30 to 40 degrees.

■ Nonsurgical

■ Radiation therapy

■ Chemotherapy

■ Surgical

— Surgical removal—craniotomy

Postoperative Care

■ Monitor for:

— ↑ ICP

— Cerebrospinal fluid leakage

— Monitor respiratory status closely

— Monitor for seizure activity

After the change of shift report, the nurse reviews her assignments. Which client should the RN assess first?

A. The elderly client receiving palliative care for heart failure who complains of constipation and nervousness

B. The adult client who is 48 hours postoperative for a colectomy and is reported to be having nausea and vomiting.

C. The middle-aged client with chronic renal failure whose urinary catheter has been draining 95 mL for 8 hours

D. The client who is 2 days postoperative for a thoracotomy and who has chest tubes, is on oxygen at 3 L/min, and has a respiratory rate of 12 breaths/min

HESI Test Question Approach			
Positive?		YES	NO
Key Words			
Rephrase			
Rule Out Choices			
A	B	C	D

A practical nurse (PN) is assigned to care for an 82-year-old client who had a total right hip replacement with cement 2 days ago. Which observation(s) should the PN immediately report to the RN? (Select all that apply.)

A. The client complains of incisional pain, rating it a 6 on a scale of 0 to 10.
B. The client has had a change in orientation to person but not to time or place.
C. Swelling and redness have developed in the client's lower left leg.
D. The PN emptied 15 mL of bloody drainage from the Jackson-Pratt drain.
E. The client's last set of vital signs was temperature 37.9° C (100.2° F), pulse 87, respiration 12, blood pressure 108/74, and O_2 saturation 93%.

HESI Test Question Approach			
Positive?		YES	NO
Key Words			
Rephrase			
Rule Out Choices			
A	B	C	D	E

The nurse is the first responder at the scene of a mass casualty incident. The nurse is tasked to triage the victims from highest to lowest priority. Arrange the victims from highest to lowest priority. All options must be used.

A. Victim A is an elder adult with agonal respirations and open head injury.
B. Victim B is a confused adult with bright red blood pulsating from a leg wound.
C. Victim C is a young adult with multiple compound fractures of the arms and legs.
D. Victim D is an adult with multiple shrapnel wounds of the face and arms complaining of abdominal pain.
E. Victim E is a sobbing adult with several minor lacerations on the face, arms, and legs.

HESI Test Question Approach			
Positive?		YES	NO
Key Words			
Rephrase			
Rule Out Choices			
A	B	C	D	E

The nurse is monitoring the status of a client recovering from a myocardial infarction. Which symptom indicates an evolving problem?

A. A steady pulse of 88 beats/min
B. Rising systolic pressure from 110 to 120 mm Hg
C. Six premature ventricular contractions/min
D. Total urine output of 110 mL/hr over 3 hours

HESI Test Question Approach			
Positive?		YES	NO
Key Words			
Rephrase			
Rule Out Choices			
A	B	C	D

Advanced Clinical Concepts

Shock

Stages of Shock

- Stage 1: Initiation
  — Early signs may include agitation and restlessness.
  — ↑ Heart rate
  — Cool, pale skin
- Stage 2: Compensatory
  — Confusion
  — Cerebral perfusion <70 mm Hg
  — Cardiac output ↓ <4 to 6 L/min
  — Systolic BP <100 mm Hg
  — ↑ Heart rate (except neurogenic)
  — ↓ Urine output (oliguria)
- Stage 3: Progressive
  — Edema
  — Severe hypotension
  — Dysrhythmia

- Weak, thready pulses
- Cold, clammy skin
- Anuria
- Stage 4: Irreversible
  - Profound hypotension
  - Unresponsive to vasopressors
  - Slowing heart rate
  - Multiple organ dysfunction syndrome (MODS)
  - Severe hypoxemia
  - Severe acidosis

Types of Shock

- Hypovolemic
  - Most common
  - Related to internal or external blood/fluid loss
- Cardiogenic
  - Pump failure
  - Results in ↓ cardiac output
- Distributive or vasogenic
  - Anaphylactic, neurogenic, and septic shock
  - Excessive vasodilation and impaired distribution of blood flow
  - Decreased arteriolar resistance
- Obstructive
  - Physical obstruction that impedes the filling and pumping of the heart

Treatment for Shock

- Correct decreased tissue perfusion and restore cardiac output.
  - Optimize oxygenation and ventilation.
  - Fluid resuscitation
- Cause of shock guides treatment
  - *Hypovolemic shock:* Volume expanding fluids for hypovolemia
  - *Cardiogenic shock:* Volume expansion may pre-cipitate pulmonary edema
  - *Distributive:* Cautious volume replacement (fluid is redistributed, not lost)
  - *Obstructive:* Physical obstruction that impeded heart filling and pumping
- Drug therapy
  - Restoration of cardiac function is based on the effect of shock on preload, afterload, and contractility.
    - Preload
      - Increase preload through crystalloids and colloids
      - Decrease preload through nitrates, diuretics, or morphine
    - Afterload
      - Increase afterload through vasopressors.
      - Decrease afterload through sodium nitroprus-side, angiotensin-converting enzyme (ACE) inhibitors, or angiotensin receptor blockers (ARBs).
    - Contractility
      - Increase contractility through dobutamine dopamine, and digoxin.
      - Decrease contractility through beta-blockers, calcium channel blockers.

A client in shock develops a mean arterial pressure (MAP) of 60 mm Hg and a heart rate of 110 beats/min. Which prescribed intervention should the nurse implement first?

A. Increase the rate of O_2 flow.
B. Obtain arterial blood gas results.
C. Insert an indwelling urinary catheter.
D. Increase the rate of intravenous (IV) fluids.

HESI Test Question Approach			
Positive?		YES	NO
Key Words			
Rephrase			
Rule Out Choices			
A	B	C	D

A client is admitted to the acute care unit with stable angina. At 7:00 AM the client has had stable vital signs and is on 2 L nasal cannula. At 10:00 AM, the client reports chest pain 6 on a scale of 1 to 10, is slightly diaphoretic and pale, blood pressure (BP) is 100/52, and respiratory rate is 24. Which action will the nurse implement first?

A. Apply 4 L of oxygen as ordered.
B. Administer a fluid bolus of 0.9 normal saline.
C. Administer the prescribed opioid for pain control.
D. Obtain a full set of vital signs including temperature.

HESI Test Question Approach			
Positive?		YES	NO
Key Words			
Rephrase			
Rule Out Choices			
A	B	C	D

A client with burn injuries has lost a significant amount of body fluid. An IV of Lactated Ringer's solution is infusing at 200 mL/hr, and the urine output for the past 8 hours is 400 mL. Which sign or symptom relates to early distributive shock?

A. A change in BP from 118/60 to 102/68
B. A change in level of consciousness from awake to restless
C. A decrease in O_2 saturation from 98% to 93%
D. A decrease in urine output over 8 hours from 400 to 240 mL

HESI Test Question Approach			
Positive?		YES	NO
Key Words			
Rephrase			
Rule Out Choices			
A	B	C	D

The Continuum of Sepsis

Systemic inflammatory response syndrome (SIRS) occurs as a response to an assortment of insults, including sepsis, ischemia, infarction, and injury. Generalized inflammation in organs remote from the initial insult characterizes the syndrome.

SIRS starts with an infection, which progresses to *bacteremia,* then *sepsis,* then *severe sepsis,* then *septic shock,* and finally to multiple organ dysfunction syndrome (MODS).

Septic shock is characterized by sepsis not responsive to fluid resuscitation.

Multiple organ dysfunction syndrome (MODS) is the failure of two or more organ systems as a result of an uncontrolled inflammatory response in critically ill clients. MODS results from SIRS. These two syndromes represent the two ends of a continuum.

The sequence of the sepsis continuum is:

1. SIRS
2. Sepsis
3. Severe sepsis
4. Septic shock
5. MODS

Nursing and Collaborative Management

- Prevention strategies
- Early recognition of subtle changes in heart rate, systolic BP, respiratory rate, oxygen saturation, urinary output, and central nervous system
- Serum lactate level
- Prevention and treatment of infection
  — Blood cultures (two sets) before starting antibiotics
  — Broad-spectrum antibiotics within 1 to 3 hours of admission or recognition of sepsis
  — Maintenance of tissue oxygenation
  — Nutritional and metabolic support
  — Support of individual failing organs

Disseminated Intravascular Coagulation (DIC)

DIC is a serious disorder of hemostasis in which clotting factors are consumed followed by subsequent bleeding. DIC is stimulated by a disease process or disorder such as septicemia, obstetric complications, malignancies, tissue trauma, transfusion reactions, burns, shock, and snakebites.

- DIC results from an initiating event with abnormal clotting in the microvasculature (↑ fibrin).
- A decrease in clotting factors and platelets ensues.
- This decrease may lead to uncontrollable hemorrhage.
- As clots break down, the clot materials (fibrin degradation products [FDPs]) are released into circulation.
- FDPs are potent anticoagulants that interfere with blood coagulation in three ways:
  — Coating platelets, interfering with platelet function
  — Interfering with thrombin, disrupting coagulation
  — Attaching to fibrinogen, interfering with clotting
- ↑ D-dimer assay test measuring the degree of fibrinolysis and ↑ fibrin split products in blood

Nursing and Collaborative Management

- Appropriate nursing interventions are essential to the client's survival.
- Astute, ongoing assessment is required.
- Early detection of bleeding, both occult and overt, must be a primary goal:
  — Assess the client for signs of external and internal bleeding.
  — Be alert for manifestations of the syndrome.

- Institution of appropriate treatment measures, which can be challenging and sometimes paradoxic:
  — Heparin infusion (early in DIC, when clots are forming)
  — Blood, FFP transfusions, and cryoprecipitate

Acute Respiratory Distress Syndrome (ARDS)

- A sudden, progressive form of acute respiratory failure that damages the alveolar capillary membrane and in-activates surfactant (causing atelectasis)
- Sepsis is the most common cause.
- Three phases:
  — Injury of exudative
  — Reparative or proliferative
  — Fibrotic
- Diagnosis
  — Refractory hypoxemia
  — A predisposing condition for ARDS within 48 hours of clinical manifestations
  — New bilateral interstitial or alveolar infiltrates on a chest radiograph (this condition on a chest x-ray is often called "whiteout" or "white lung")
  — Alveolar capillary membrane damage with interstitial and alveolar edema
  — Pulmonary artery occlusion pressure (PAOP) of 18 mm Hg or less (normal) and no evidence of heart failure
- As ARDS progresses, it is associated with profound respiratory distress requiring endotracheal intubation and positive pressure ventilation (PPV).

Nursing Assessment

- Hypoxemia
- Dyspnea
- Tachypnea
- Scattered crackles
- Increased work of breathing
- Respiratory alkalosis (early sign—hyperventilation)
- Respiratory acidosis (later sign—muscle fatigue)
- Pleural effusions
- Decreased cardiac output
- Cyanosis

Nursing and Collaborative Management

- Overall goals for a client with ARDS
  — Pao_2 of at least 60 mm Hg
  — Adequate lung ventilation to maintain normal pH
- Goals for a client recovering from ARDS
  — Pao_2 within normal limits for age or baseline values on room air
  — Sao_2 >90%
  — Patent airway
  — Clear lungs on auscultation
- Oxygen to correct hypoxemia
- Positive pressure ventilation
- Positive end-expiratory pressure (PEEP)
  — A ventilatory option that creates positive pressure at end exhalation and restores functional residual capacity (FRC) and opens collapsed alveoli
- Prone position

Delirium

- An acute state of temporary confusion, difficulty concentrating, and clouded sensorium
- The most frequent complication in older, hospitalized adults
- May be a symptom of a serious medical illness
- Risk factors
  - Sleep deprivation, advanced age or vision, and hearing impairment
  - Use of opioids and/or corticosteroids
  - Drug or alcohol abuse
  - Urinary tract infection, fluid and electrolyte imbalance
  - Unscheduled surgery, postoperative, intensive care unit, or emergent delirium

Nursing and Collaborative Management

- Prevention and early recognition
- Protect the client from harm.
- Provide a low-stimulation environment (calm).
- Approach the client slowly and from the front.
- Reorient the client and communicate with simple statements.
- Monitor neurological status on an ongoing basis.
- Consider management with neuroleptic drugs (e.g., haloperidol).
- Encourage family visibility and support.

A client recovering from ARDS is awake and alert, has residual fatigue and generalized weakness. His current vital signs are heart rate 83, blood pressure 104/64, respiratory rate 25, Spo₂ on 2 L/min nasal oxygen air is 92%. Which vital sign value should unlicensed assistive personnel report immediately to the nurse?

A. Heart rate of 88 beats per minute
B. Blood pressure of 104/64 mm Hg
C. Respiratory rate of 25 breaths per minute
D. Spo₂ 92%

HESI Test Question Approach			
Positive?		**YES**	**NO**
Key Words			
Rephrase			
Rule Out Choices			
A	B	C	D

An elderly client's vital signs are 103° F (39.6° C), heart rate 109, respiratory rate 37, blood pressure 86/42. After an infusion of 1.5 L of 0.9 Normal Saline IV there are few changes in vital signs. The nurse assesses the client and develops a plan of care based on which client disease or disorder?

A. Septic shock
B. Multiple organ failure
C. Acute respiratory distress syndrome
D. Systemic inflammatory response syndrome

HESI Test Question Approach			
Positive?		**YES**	**NO**
Key Words			
Rephrase			
Rule Out Choices			
A	B	C	D

A 22-year-old client is admitted through the emergency department with a 2-day history of cough, fever, and fatigue. The medical history is positive for type I diabetes and recent upper respiratory infection. Vital signs are heart rate 109, blood pressure 102/58, respiratory rate 24, temperature 104° F (40° C), and SpO_2 of 92% on 2 L nasal cannula. Which prescription has the highest priority in this client's care?

A. Initiate large bore IV access.
B. Draw two sets of blood cultures.
C. Administer the ordered IV antibiotics.
D. Draw serum lactate and glucose levels.

HESI Test Question Approach			
Positive?		YES	NO
Key Words			
Rephrase			
Rule Out Choices			
A	B	C	D

A client with a history of uterine fibroids had a cesarean delivery 12 hours earlier and delivered healthy twin girls. At shift change, the nurse assesses the client and notes shortness of breath, cool extremities, and oozing of blood from the incision site. Based on the client's presentation, what action has the highest priority?

A. Assess the client's temperature.
B. Notify the health care provider.
C. Clean the blood from the incision site.
D. Draw labs for prothrombin time, partial prothrombin time, fibrinogen, and complete blood count.

HESI Test Question Approach			
Positive?		YES	NO
Key Words			
Rephrase			
Rule Out Choices			
A	B	C	D

Life Support

- Cardiac arrest is the most common event requiring cardiopulmonary resuscitation (CPR).
- C-A-B—**C**hest compressions–**A**irway–**B**reathing
  - Emphasis is on high-quality chest compressions.
  - Push hard and push fast
  - Depth of 2 inches; be sure to let chest recoil after each compression
  - Adult 100 compressions/min
- In-hospital cardiac arrest
  - Initiate CPR with basic cardiac life support (BCLS) guidelines, moving to advanced cardiac life support (ACLS) guidelines.
  - Determine unresponsiveness.
  - Activate emergency response or cardiac arrest team.
  - Obtain automatic external defibrillator (AED) and/or emergency crash cart with defibrillator (do not leave client).
- If pulse is not identified with 10 seconds:
  - Initiate chest compressions.
  - After 30 compressions, open airway with head-tilt chin lift, and ventilate with bag-valve mask; provide 2 breaths each over 1 second.
  - Maintain compressions-to-breaths ratio of 30:2.
  - Once the AED or defibrillator arrives, apply "quick look" paddles or AED to determine whether defibrillation is necessary; defibrillate as indicated, following hospital policies and procedures.

— Resume CPR; begin with compression immediately after defibrillation.

— Prepare to administer epinephrine and follow hospital protocols as indicated.

CPR and Choking Basics: Neonates and Children 1 to 8 Years

- Indications for CPR in children are different from those in adults.
  - *Neonates and infants:* Hypoxia, hypoglycemia, hypothermia, acidosis, hypercoagulability
  - *Children:* Respiratory arrest, prolonged hypoxemia secondary to respiratory insult or shock, including septic shock
- Guidelines vary based on child's age.
- If no response occurs, call a "code," or cardiac arrest, to initiate response of cardiac arrest team.
  - Obtain AED or emergency crash cart with defibrillator.
  - Check for pulse:
    - Infant <1 year: brachial pulse
    - Children 1 year to puberty: carotid or femoral
- Compressions (begin within 10 seconds)
  - *Infants (most):* Compressions cover at least one third of the anterior/posterior diameter of the chest to a depth of 1.5 inches
  - *Children (most):* Compressions cover at least one third of the anterior/posterior diameter of the chest to a depth of 2 inches
  - *If one rescuer:* 30 compressions to 2 breaths
  - *If two rescuers:* 15 compressions to 2 breath
- Deliver each breath over 1 second (avoid excessive ventilation—will cause gastric inflation).
- Minimize interruption in compressions.
- Allow full chest recoil.

For up-to-date information on foreign body obstructed airway and CPR, see the American Heart Association website for CPR guidelines: www.heart.org/HEARTORG/

The cardiac monitor alarms, and the nurse arrives to find the 59-year-old client slumped in the chair. Place the nurse's actions in order of priority for this client from first to last.
A. Activate the code team and obtain defibrillator.
B. Determine unresponsiveness.
C. Assess the cardiac rhythm using the "quick look" paddles.
D. Assess for a pulse (carotid).
E. Open airway and give two rescue breaths by bag-valve mask.
F. Move the client to a flat position in bed or on the floor.
G. Begin compressions.

HESI Test Question Approach			
Positive?		YES	NO
Key Words			
Rephrase			
Rule Out Choices			
A	B	C	D	E	F	G

Disaster Management

- The nurse is an active team member in the event of biological, chemical, radioactive, mass trauma, and natural disasters.
- The nurse plays a role at all three levels of disaster management.

Preparedness, Response, Recovery

- Levels of prevention in disaster management
  - *Primary:* Planning, training, educating personnel and the public
  - *Secondary:* Triage, treatment, shelter supervision
  - *Tertiary:* Follow-up, recovery assistance, prevention of future disasters

Triage

The goal of triage is to maximize the number of survivors by sorting the injured as treatable and untreatable, using the criteria of potential for survival and availability of resources.

- Color-coded system (in order of priority)
  - *Red:* life threatening, need immediate intervention
  - *Yellow:* injuries with systemic effects and complications
  - *Green:* minor injuries, no systemic complications
  - *Black:* dying or deceased—catastrophic injuries
- START (**S**imple **T**riage **A**nd **R**apid **T**reatment) method
- Identify the walking wounded; move them to an area where they can be evaluated later
- Three-step evaluation of others, done one at a time:
  - Assess RESPIRATIONS
  - Assess CIRCULATION
  - Assess MENTAL STATUS

Several clients present to the triage nurse in the emergency department (ED). Which client should the nurse ask the health care provider to see first?

A. A teary 19-year-old client with a temperature of 38.2° C (100.8° F) who has had vomiting and watery diarrhea five times in 3 hours

B. A middle-aged client who has had a sore throat, swollen lymph nodes, and cough for 2 days and who had received the flu vaccine

C. A 40-year-old client brought to the ED by her co-workers, who has had a severe headache, vomiting, and a stiff neck for 48 hours

D. A 60-year-old client limping on a swollen ankle and complaining of ankle pain who has been self-medicating with oxycodone/acetaminophen

HESI Test Question Approach		
Positive?	**YES**	**NO**
Key Words		
Rephrase		
Rule Out Choices		
A	**B**	**C**	**D**

The nurse is assessing clients at the site of a community disaster. Using the color-code system for triage, which client should the nurse tag with a red code?

A. A client with a large head injury that is bleeding, an open chest wound, cyanotic skin, no capillary refill, and agonal respirations
B. A client with bruising and swelling of the right forearm, assorted lacerations to the face and neck, dry skin, normal capillary refill, and a respiratory rate of 18
C. A client with scratches and scrapes to the head and face who is limping and helping other clients at the scene
D. A client with an open wound to the abdomen, and a deformed right femur, pulse 125, delayed capillary refill, respiratory rate 32, who is moaning

HESI Test Question Approach			
Positive?		YES	NO
Key Words			
Rephrase			
Rule Out Choices			
A	B	C	D

Bioterrorism

Review exposure information, assessment findings, and treatment for various agents:
- Biological
- Chemical
- Radiation

Exam questions may deal with disasters and bioterrorism as they affect the individual victim, families, and the community.

The nurse is completing discharge teaching for a group of postal employees who have been exposed to a powder form of anthrax. Which instruction has the highest priority?

A. Begin the prescribed antibiotics and continue for 60 days.
B. Watch for symptoms of anthrax for the next 7 days.
C. Make arrangements to be vaccinated for anthrax.
D. Explain to family members that anthrax is not contagious.

HESI Test Question Approach			
Positive?		YES	NO
Key Words			
Rephrase			
Rule Out Choices			
A	B	C	D

The emergency department nurse is assessing a client with suspected smallpox exposure after a subway terror attack with a biological agent. To mitigate the exposure risk to other people, the nurse will place the client on which type of transmission precautions? Select all that apply.

A. Airborne
B. Contact
C. Aplastic
D. Droplet
E. Standard

HESI Test Question Approach				
Positive?			YES	NO
Key Words				
Rephrase				
Rule Out Choices				
A	B	C	D	E

5 Oxygenation, Ventilation, Transportation, and Perfusion

A client who is 1 day postoperative from a left pneumonectomy is lying on his right side with the head of the bed (HOB) elevated 10 degrees. The nurse assesses his respiratory rate at 32 breaths/min. What action should the nurse take first?
A. Further elevate HOB.
B. Assist the client into the supine position.
C. Measure the client's O_2 saturation.
D. Administer intravenous (IV) PRN (as needed) morphine.

HESI Test Question Approach			
Positive?		YES	NO
Key Words			
Rephrase			
Rule Out Choices			
A	B	C	D

Chest Tube and Water or Dry Seal Management

- Chest tubes are inserted into the pleural space to remove air and fluid and to allow the lung to reexpand.
- A chest collection drainage system has three compartments or chambers.
  — Collection chamber:
    - Air and fluid are collected from the pleural or mediastinal space.
    - Fluid remains and air is vented to the second compartment, the water seal chamber.
  — Water-seal chamber:
    - This chamber contains 2 cm of water, which prevents backflow and acts as a one-way valve.
    - Fluctuations in the water level are known as "tidaling"; fluid should move upward with each inspiration and downward with each expiration.
  — Suction control chamber:
    - Water suction uses 20 cm of water to aid in draining air or fluid from the chest.
    - Dry suction provides a safe and effective level of vacuum by continuously balancing the forces of suction and atmosphere.

Nursing and Collaborative Management

- Keep all tubing coiled loosely below chest level, with connections tight and taped.
- Monitor the fluid drainage and mark the time of measurement and the fluid level; notify healthcare provider if there is >100 mL/hr drainage.
- Observe for air bubbling in the water-seal chamber and fluctuations (tidaling).
- Replace the unit when full.
- Do not routinely clamp chest tubes; milking or stripping chest tubes is not recommended.

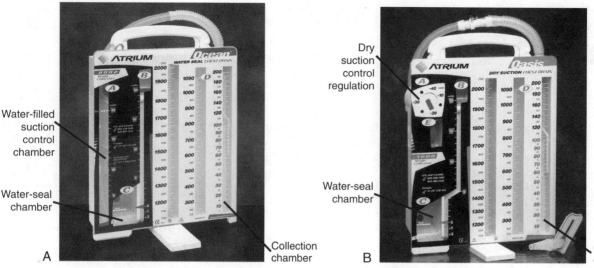

Figure 5-1   Chest drainage unit. Both units have three chambers: (1) collection chamber; (2) water-seal chamber; and (3) suction control chamber. The suction control chamber requires a connection to a wall suction source that is dialed to the prescribed suction. **A,** Water suction. This unit uses water in the suction control chamber to control the wall suction pressure. **B,** Dry suction. This unit controls wall suction by using a regulator control dial. (From Lewis, S. L., et al (2014). *Medical-surgical nursing: Assessment and management of clinical problems* (9th ed.). St Louis: Mosby.)

- If the chest tube is accidentally dislodged, the nurse should:
  — Cover the area with a dry, sterile dressing
  — If an air leak is noted, tape the dressing on three sides only; this allows air to escape and prevents the formation of a tension pneumothorax
  — Notify the healthcare provider

Pneumonia

Pneumonia results in inflammation of lung tissue, causing consolidation of exudate.
- Etiology
  — Bacterial (gram-negative is the most severe), viral, fungal (rare), or aspiration
  — Community acquired (CAP) or hospital acquired (HAP)
  — Ventilator-associated pneumonia (VAP)
- Risk factors
  — Age >65 years or residents in long-term care
  — Recent surgery (abdominal, thoracic)
  — Altered consciousness: alcoholism, head injury, seizures, anesthesia, drug overdose, cerebrovascular accident
  — Prolonged immobility
- Prevention
  — Pneumovax vaccine for at risk or age >65 years and a second vaccine if more than 5 years have passed since the initial vaccine
  — Seasonal influenza vaccines yearly
  — VAP practice bundles
    • Meticulous hand hygiene
    • Closed ventilator system and suction

- HOB elevation 30 to 45 degrees
- Oral care before intubation and routinely per facility protocol
- Drain all water that collects in the ventilator tubing
- Suction only as needed with aseptic technique
- Use routine peptic ulcer prophylaxis

The spouse of a 94-year-old client reports to the home health nurse that his wife has become increasingly confused over the past few days and has developed a cough. Which assessment should the nurse perform first?
A. Jugular vein distention
B. Skin turgor
C. Oxygen saturation
D. Pupillary response to light

HESI Test Question Approach

Positive?		YES	NO
Key Words			
Rephrase			
Rule Out Choices			
A	B	C	D

The nurse is orienting a graduate nurse (GN) caring for a client dependent on the ventilator. Which action by the GN demonstrates understanding of ventilator-associated pneumonia (VAP) care? (Select all that apply.)
A. Changes ventilator tubing every 72 hours
B. Performs oral care every 2 hours
C. Elevates the HOB to 60 degrees
D. Performs suction with 5 mL of saline
E. Does hand hygiene before and after care

HESI Test Question Approach

Positive?			YES	NO
Key Words				
Rephrase				
Rule Out Choices				
A	B	C	D	E

Nursing Assessment

- Tachypnea
- Productive cough
- Pleuritic pain
- Fever of abrupt onset
- Dyspnea
- Cyanosis
- Mental status changes
- Crackles, decreased breath sounds
- Dullness on percussion
- ABGs indicative of hypoxemia

Nursing and Collaborative Management

- Hand washing to reduce cross-contamination
- Blood cultures and sputum cultures
- Isolation if prescribed
- Administer and encourage fluids if not contraindicated.
- Administer antipyretics.
- Manage pain.
- Monitor oxygen saturation and administer oxygen as appropriate (humidified to loosen secretions).
- Teach coughing, turning and deep breathing techniques.
- Bronchial hygiene: Encourage use of incentive spirometry.

Antiinfectives
- — Penicillins
  - Semisynthetic penicillins
  - Oxacillin
- — Antipseudomonal penicillins
  - Piperacillin sodium
- — Tetracyclines
- — Aminoglycosides
  - Gentamicin sulfate
- — Cephalosporins
  - Ceftriaxone sodium
- — Macrolides
  - Clarithromycin (Biaxin)
- — Fluoroquinolones
  - Ciprofloxacin (Cipro)

Chronic Airflow Limitation (CAL)

- Asthma—a reversible disease
- Chronic obstructive pulmonary disease (COPD)—a chronic progressive disease
  - — Emphysema
  - — Chronic bronchitis

Etiology and Precipitating Factors for COPD

- Cigarette smoking
- Environmental/occupational exposure
- Genetic predisposition

Chronic Bronchitis

- Pathophysiology
  - — Chronic sputum with cough production on a daily basis for a minimum of 3 months/year
  - — Chronic hypoxemia/cor pulmonale
  - — Increased mucus production
  - — Increased bronchial wall thickness (obstructs air flow)
  - — Exacerbations usually due to infection
  - — Increased CO_2 retention/acidemia
  - — Reduced responsiveness of respiratory center to hypoxemic stimuli
  - — ↑ CO_2 retention/acidemia
  - — Reduced responsiveness of respiratory center to hypoxemic stimuli

Emphysema

- Abnormal enlargement of the air spaces distal to the terminal alveolar walls
- Increased dyspnea/work of breathing
  - — Reduced gas exchange surface area
  - — Increased air trapping (increased anterior-posterior diameter)
  - — Decreased capillary network
  - — Increased work/increased O_2 consumption

Nursing Assessment: COPD

- Inspection
  - Bronchitis
    - Right-sided heart failure
    - Cyanosis distended neck veins
  - Emphysema
    - Pursed-lip breathing
    - Noncyanotic, thin
  - Auscultation
    - Crackles
    - Rhonchi
    - Expiratory wheezes
  - Emphysema
    - Distant breath sounds
    - Quiet breath sounds
    - Wheezes

Nursing and Collaborative Management: COPD

- Lowest O_2 to prevent CO_2 retention
  - Take particular care not to abolish the hypoxic drive needed for effective breathing if the client has COPD and is known to retain CO_2.
  - Obtain parameters for acceptable O_2 saturation levels.
- Monitor for signs and symptoms (S/S) of fluid overload.
- Baseline ABGs for CO_2 retainers
- Teach the client pursed-lip breathing.
- Orthopneic position

An elderly man comes to the emergency department (ED) complaining of shortness of breath. The healthcare provider (HCP) determines that the client has pneumonia. The client's condition deteriorates in the ED, and he now has impending respiratory failure. Which set of arterial blood gas (ABG) values demonstrates acute respiratory failure?

A. pH–7.30 P_{CO_2}–52 P_{O_2}–56 H_{CO_3}–26
B. pH–7.35 P_{CO_2}–44 P_{O_2}–86 H_{CO_3}–28
C. pH–7.35 P_{CO_2}–62 P_{O_2}–66 H_{CO_3}–31
D. pH–7.30 P_{CO_2}–39 P_{O_2}–88 H_{CO_3}–22

HESI Test Question Approach		
Positive?	**YES**	**NO**
Key Words		
Rephrase		
Rule Out Choices		
A	**B**	**C** **D**

Reactive Airway Disease

Asthma

Asthma is a reversible inflammatory disorder of the airways characterized by an exaggerated bronchoconstrictor response to a wide variety of stimuli.

- Allergens
- Environmental irritants
- Cold air
- Exercise
- β-blockers
- Respiratory infection
- Emotional stress
- Reflux esophagitis

Drug Therapy for Asthma and COPD
Bronchodilators
- Short-acting inhaled β_2-adrenergic agonists
- Long-acting inhaled β_2-adrenergic agonists
- Long-acting oral β_2-adrenergic agonists
- Theophylline (Theolair, Uniphyl)
- Anticholinergics (inhaled)

β_2-Adrenergic Agonists
Inhaled: Short Acting
- Metaproterenol: nebulizer, oral tablets, elixir, metered-dose inhaler (MDI)
- Salbutamol sulfate (Albuterol, Proventil, Apo-Salvent, Ventolin HFA, Volmax): nebulizer, MDI, oral tablets, Rotahaler
- Levalbuterol (Xopenex, Xopenex HFA): nebulizer, MDI
- Terbutaline (Bricanyl, Brethine): oral tablets, nebulizer, subcutaneous, MDI
- Bitolterol (Tornalate): MDI, nebulizer

Inhaled: Long Acting
- Salmeterol xinafoate (Serevent): dry powder inhaler (DPI)
- Formoterol fumarate (Foradil): DPI

Immediate Acting
- Epinephrine hydrochloride (Adrenalin chloride): (1:1000) subcutaneous

Corticosteroids
- Hydrocortisone (Solu-Cortef): IV
- Methylprednisolone (Solu-Medrol): IV
- Prednisone: oral
- Beclomethasone dipropionate (Gen-Beclo AQ Vanceril, Beclovent, Vanceril DS, Qvar): inhaler
- Triamcinolone acetonide (Nasacort AQ Azmacort): inhaler
- Fluticasone propionate (Flonase, Flovent HFA): inhaler
- Budesonide (Pulmicort Turbuhaler): inhaler
- Mometasone furoate monohydrate (Nasonex): inhaler

Anticholinergics
- Short-acting ipratropium bromide (Atrovent): nebulizer, MDI
- Long-acting tiotropium (Spiriva): DPI
- Mast cell stabilizers: nedocromil sodium

IgE Antagonist
- Omalizumab (Xolair): subcutaneous injection

Leukotriene Modifiers
- Leukotriene receptor blockers
  — Zafirlukast (Accolate) oral tablets
  — Montelukast sodium (Singulair) oral tablets, chewable tablets, oral granules
- Leukotriene inhibitor
  — Zileuton (Zyflo) oral tablets

Methylxanthines
- Aminophylline as an IV agent is rarely used; available as oral, rectal, injectable, and topical.
- Oral: Elixophyllin, Quibron, Slo-bid

Combination Agents
- Ipratropium and salbutamol (Combivent): MDI, nebulizer
- Fluticasone propionate/salmeterol (Advair Diskus): DPI

Nursing Assessment
- Dyspnea, wheezing, chest tightness
- Assess precipitating factors
- Medication history

Nursing and Collaborative Management
- Monitor respirations and assess breath sounds
- Monitor oxygen saturation
- Monitor mental status
- Chest physiotherapy
- Assess peripheral pulses and warmth and color of extremities
- Position for maximum ventilation
- Encourage slow, pursed-lip breathing
- Encourage abdominal breathing
- Administer humidified oxygen therapy
- Provide education on peak flow meter monitoring, importance of medication compliance, and trigger avoidance

The nurse palpates a crackling sensation of the skin around the insertion site of a chest tube in a client who has had thoracic surgery. What action should the nurse take?

A. Return the client to surgery.
B. Prepare for insertion of a larger chest tube.
C. Increase the water-seal suction pressure.
D. Continue to monitor the insertion site.

The nurse is preparing to administer a Mantoux (PPD—purified protein derivative) test to a client who is entering nursing school. Which action by the nurse is of highest priority?

A. Prepare 0.1-mL solution per tuberculin syringe.
B. Assess the skin condition on the forearm.
C. Teach the client about positive findings.
D. Inquire about bacillus Calmette-Guérin (BCG) vaccine history.

HESI Test Question Approach			
Positive?		YES	NO
Key Words			
Rephrase			
Rule Out Choices			
A	B	C	D

HESI Test Question Approach			
Positive?		YES	NO
Key Words			
Rephrase			
Rule Out Choices			
A	B	C	D

Pulmonary Tuberculosis (TB)

TB is a communicable lung disease caused by the bacillus *Mycobacterium tuberculosis* or the tubercle bacillus, an acid-fast organism that is spread by airborne transmission.

Resurgence of TB

- Related to immunocompromised states
- Multidrug-resistant TB (MDR-TB)
- Rifampin
- Isoniazid
- Seen disproportionately in poor, underserved, and minorities

Nursing Assessment

- Low-grade fever
- Pallor
- Chills
- Night sweats
- Easy fatigability
- Anorexia
- Weight loss

Nursing and Collaborative Management

- Diagnosis with acid amplification test (NAAT), QuantiFERON-TB, or purified protein derivative (PPD)
- Airborne precautions isolation
- Single-occupancy room with negative pressure and airflow of 6 to 12 exchanges per hour
- Wear high-efficiency particulate air (HEPA) masks.
- Teach client to cover the nose and mouth with paper tissues whenever coughing, sneezing, or producing sputum.
- Sputum specimens are collected at 2- to 4-week intervals with a return to work after three negative specimens in a row are achieved.
- Emphasize careful hand washing after handling sputum and soiled tissues.
- If client needs to be out of the negative-pressure room, he or she must wear a standard isolation mask to prevent exposure to others.
- Medication regimen
  - First-line therapy: isoniazid (INH), rifampin, and pyrazinamide added for the first 2 months, which potentially shortens therapy to 6 months
  - Isoniazid (INH therapy)
  - Pyridoxine (vitamin B_6)
  - Rifampin (Rifadin, Rofact)
  - Pyrazinamide
  - With or without streptomycin and ethambutol (Etibi)
  - Take as prescribed (6 to 24 months)
- Teach client medication side effects.

TB Drugs and Side Effects

First-Line Drugs

First-line drugs are bacteriocidal against rapidly dividing cells and/or against semidormant bacteria.

- Isoniazid (INH): clinical hepatitis, fulminant hepatitis, peripheral neurotoxicity
- Rifampin (Rifadin, Rofact): cutaneous reactions, gastrointestinal (GI) disturbance (nausea, anorexia, abdominal pain), flulike syndrome, hepatotoxicity, immunological reactions, orange discoloration of bodily fluids (sputum, urine, sweat, tears)
- Ethambutol hydrochloride (Myambutol Etibi): retrobulbar neuritis (decreased red-green color discrimination), skin rash
- Rifabutin (Mycobutin): hematologic toxicity, GI symptoms, polyarthralgia, pseudojaundice, orange discoloration of bodily fluids
- Pyrazinamide (PZA): hepatotoxicity, GI symptoms (nausea, vomiting), polyarthralgia, skin rash, hyperuricemia, dermatitis

Second-Line Drugs

Second-line drugs are bactericidal and/or bacteriostatic and/or inhibit cell wall synthesis.

- Cycloserine (Seromycin): central nervous system effects; given with pyridoxine to prevent neurotoxic effects
- Ethionamide (Trecator): hepatotoxicity, neurotoxicity, GI effects (metallic taste, nausea, vomiting), endocrine effects (hypothyroidism, impotence)
- Streptomycin sulfate: ototoxicity, neurotoxicity, nephrotoxicity
- Amikacin sulfate and kanamycin: ototoxicity, nephrotoxicity
- Para-aminosalicylic acid (PAS): hepatotoxicity, GI distress, malabsorption syndrome, coagulopathy
- Fluoroquinolones (levofloxacin [Levaquin], moxifloxacin hydrochloride [Avelox, Vigamox], gatifloxacin [Tequin]): GI disturbances, neurological effects (dizziness, headaches), rash

Pulmonary Embolus

Any substance can cause an embolism. Typically, a blood clot enters the venous circulation and lodges in the pulmonary vasculature.

Risk Factors for Venous Thromboembolism Leading to Pulmonary Embolism

- Prolonged immobility
- Central venous catheters
- Surgery
- Obesity
- Advancing age
- Conditions that increase blood clotting
- History of thromboembolism
- Smoking, birth control pills, pregnancy

Signs and Symptoms

- Dyspnea, tachypnea, tachycardia
- Apprehension, restlessness, feeling of impending doom
- Cough, hemoptysis, diaphoresis
- Crackles, pleural friction rub
- Decreased arterial oxygen saturation (SaO_2), respiratory alkalosis, then respiratory acidosis
- Sharp, stabbing chest pain
- Clear lung sounds or crackles
- Pleural friction rub
- Tachycardia
- S3 or S4 heart sound
- Diaphoresis
- Low-grade fever
- ECG-abnormal, nonspecific, and transient; T-wave and ST-segment changes
- Decreased arterial oxygen saturation (SaO_2); respiratory alkalosis, then respiratory acidosis
- Elevated D-dimer level
- Diagnosed by findings: spiral computed tomography (CT) scans, transesophageal echocardiography (TEE)

Nursing and Collaborative Management
Prevention
- Range-of-motion exercises
- Ambulate and turn.
- Avoid popliteal pressure.
- Use antiembolism and pneumatic compression stockings.
- Administer prescribed prophylactic low-dose anticoagulant and antiplatelet drugs.
- Administer stool softeners.
- Teach client and family about precautions.
- Encourage client to stop smoking.
- Encourage regular physical activity.
- Encourage weight loss and fluid intake as appropriate.
- Avoid crossing legs and restrictive clothing.
- Avoid straining, breath-holding.

Acute Management
- Oxygen therapy
- Monitor ABG studies, telemetry, and pulse oximetry.
- Assess vital signs, lung sounds, and cardiac and respiratory status.
- Anticoagulants are used to prevent embolus enlargement and the formation of new clots; use with caution with active bleeding, stroke, and recent trauma.
- Heparin is usually used unless the pulmonary embolism (PE) is massive or occurs with hemodynamic instability
- Alteplase (Activase, tPA Cathflo), fibrinolytic drugs
  — Therapeutic PTT; *activated partial thromboplastin time (aPTT)* values usually range from 1.5 to 2.5
  — Both heparin and fibrinolytic drugs are high-alert drugs.
  — Monitor for bleeding.
- Embolectomy
- Inferior vena cava filtration with placement of a vena cava filter

Hematological Problems

Anemia

- Etiology
  - Decreased erythrocyte production
  - Decreased hemoglobin synthesis
  - Iron deficiency anemia
  - Defective DNA synthesis
  - Vitamin B_{12} deficiency
  - Folic acid deficiency
  - Decreased number of erythrocyte precursors
  - Aplastic anemia
  - Chronic diseases or disorders
  - Chemotherapy
  - Blood loss
    - Acute
    - Chronic (gastritis, hemorrhoids)
  - Trauma
  - Blood vessel rupture
  - Menorrhagia

Nursing Assessment

- Pallor
- Fatigue
- Exercise intolerance
- Tachycardia
- Dyspnea
- Complete blood count
- Assess for risk factors.
- Diet low in iron, vitamin B_{12} deficiency, history of bleeding, long-term NSAID use
- Hgb <100 mmol/L (10g/dL), Hct <0.36 volume fraction (36%), RBCs <4×10^{12}/L

Nursing and Collaborative Management

- Treatment of underlying pathology
- Administer blood products as prescribed.
- Encourage diet high in iron-rich foods, folic acid, vitamin B_{12}, vitamin B_6, amino acids, and vitamin C.
- Give parenteral iron via Z-track technique.

The charge nurse is planning client assignments for the unit. The collaborative care team consists of a registered nurse (RN), a practical nurse (PN), and unlicensed assistive personnel (UAP). Which client(s) should be assigned to the RN? (Select all that apply.)

A. A client pending a blood transfusion for chronic gastrointestinal bleeding with an Hgb 70 g/L (7.0 mg/dL)

B. A client with pernicious anemia who is pending vitamin B_{12} injection

C. A client with resolving sickle cell crisis pending IV fluid conversion to saline lock

D. A client with a pressure ulcer who has been prescribed negative pressure (wound VAC) care

E. A client who received two blood transfusions yesterday and is pending AM care

HESI Test Question Approach		
Positive?	**YES**	**NO**
Key Words		
Rephrase		
Rule Out Choices		
A	B	C	D	E

Blood Transfusions

Blood Groups and Types

- ABO system includes A, B, O, and AB blood types.
- Rh factor is an antigenic substance in the erythrocytes.
- If blood is mismatched during transfusion, a transfusion reaction occurs.
  — Transfusion reaction is an antigen-antibody reaction.
  — It can range from a mild response to severe anaphylactic shock.

Types of Reactions

- Acute hemolytic
- Febrile, nonhemolytic (most common)
- Mild allergic
- Anaphylactic
- Delayed hemolytic

Types of Blood Products

- Red blood cells (RBCs)
  — Packed RBCs (PRBCs)
  — Autologous PRBCs
  — Washed RBCs
  — Frozen RBCs
  — Leukocyte-poor RBCs
  — RBC units with high number of reticulocytes (young RBCs)
- Other cellular components
  — Platelets
  — Granulocytes
- Plasma components
  — Fresh frozen plasma (FFP)
  — Cryoprecipitate
  — Serum albumin
  — Plasma protein fraction (PPF)
  — Immune serum globulin

Nursing and Collaborative Management

- Perform assessment before, during, and after transfusion, including the IV site.
- Two identifiers
- Confirm informed consent.
- Identify the compatibility.
- Initiate a transfusion slowly, then maintain the infusion rate.
  — 1 unit of PRBCs is transfused in 2 to 4 hours.

A client who is receiving a transfusion of packed red blood cells has an inflamed IV site. What action should the nurse take?

A. Double-check the blood type of the transfusing unit of blood with another nurse.
B. Discontinue the transfusion and send the remaining blood and tubing to the lab.
C. Immediately start a new IV at another site and resume the transfusion at the new site.
D. Continue to monitor the site for signs of infection and notify the healthcare provider.

HESI Test Question Approach				
Positive?			YES	NO
Key Words				
Rephrase				
Rule Out Choices				
A	B		C	D

Hypertension (HTN)

- Persistent BP elevation >140/90 mm Hg
- Risk factors
  - Nonmodifiable: family history, gender, age, ethnicity
  - Modifiable: use of alcohol, tobacco, caffeine; sedentary lifestyle; obesity

Medications

- Diuretics
  - Thiazides, metolazone (Zaroxolyn)
- Antihypertensives
  - Prazosin hydrochloride (Minipress), Atenolol (Tenormin), Clonidine (Catapres)
- Angiotensin-converting enzyme (ACE) inhibitors
  - Lisinopril (Zestril)
- Calcium channel blockers
  - Diltiazem hydrochloride (Cardizem)

HTN Education

- The number one cause of stroke (cerebrovascular accident [CVA]) is nonadherence to antihypertensive medications.

The charge nurse is planning client assignments for the unit. The collaborative care team consists of an RN, a PN, and a UAP. Which client (s) should be assigned to the PN? (Select all that apply.)

A. A client with a history of heart failure who has had no urinary output for the past 2 hours
B. A client with a history of angina who requires his morning medications
C. A client recently admitted and anticipating oral antibiotics for cellulitis
D. A client with a history of Raynaud syndrome who is pending a dressing change
E. A client with an acute deep vein thrombosis who requires a heparin hourly infusion

HESI Test Question Approach					
Positive?				YES	NO
Key Words					
Rephrase					
Rule Out Choices					
A	B		C	D	E

Coronary Artery Disease (CAD)

- Prevalent etiologies of CAD
  — Atherosclerosis: Partially or completely blocked coronary arteries
  — Coronary vasospasm
  — Microvascular angina
- CAD results in ischemia and infarction of myocardial tissue.
- Left anterior descending artery (LAD) is most commonly affected.
- Highly sensitive C-reactive protein (hsCRP)

CAD is one of the leading causes of morbidity and mortality among adults in Canada and remains the number one health problem in the United States.

Reduction of Risk Factors

- Smoking cessation
- Weight loss, DASH (Dietary Approaches to Stop Hypertension) to diet
- Lowering cholesterol levels
- Glycemic control
- Stress reduction
- Medication compliance: antihypertensives, antilipidemics
- Increase activity/exercise

Angina

- Stable angina: predictable, subsides with rest
- Unstable angina: unpredictable, may not subside with rest or nitroglycerin
- Prinzmetal (variant) angina: vasospasm etiology, occurs at rest and may be precipitated by smoking or other substance
- May radiate to either arm and to shoulder, jaw, neck, or epigastric area
- Other signs/symptoms: dyspnea, tachycardia, palpitations, nausea and vomiting, dyspepsia, fatigue, diaphoresis, pallor, syncope
- Often precipitated by exercise, cold exposure, heavy meal, stress, intercourse

Diet Therapy

- Dietary modification: DASH
- Goal is to reduce serum cholesterol and serum triglycerides.
- Maintain ideal body weight.
- Daily cholesterol intake should be restricted to <200 mg/day.

Drug Classes for Angina Management

- Antiplatelet agents
- Acetylsalicylic acid (ASA, aspirin)
- Clopidogrel (Plavix)
- GPIIb/IIIa inhibitor (potent platelet inhibitors): eptifibatide (Integrilin)
- Beta-blockers
  — Atenolol (Tenormin)
  — Metoprolol tartrate (Lopressor, Betaloc)

- Nitrates
  — Nitroglycerin
  — Isosorbide dinitrate
  — Sodium nitroprusside
- Calcium channel blockers
  — Diltiazem (Cardizem)
  — Verapamil hydrochloride
- Thrombolytics
  — Alteplase (recombinant t-PA; Activase, Cathflo)
  — Reteplase (Retavase)
  — Tenecteplase (TNKase)
  — Streptokinase (Streptase)
- Anticoagulants
  — Unfractionated heparin
  — Low-molecular-weight heparin (LMWH) (enoxaparin sodium [Lovenox])
- ACE inhibitors
  — Captopril (Capoten)
  — Enalapril sodium (Vasotec)
  — Benazepril hydrochloride (Lotensin)
- Analgesics
  — Morphine sulfate

Cholesterol-Lowering Drugs

These drugs may be initiated if dietary modification is unsuccessful.

- Atorvastatin calcium (Lipitor)
- Lovastatin (Mevacor)
- Pravastatin sodium (Pravasa; Pravachol)
- Rosuvastatin calcium (Crestor)
- Simvastatin (Zocor)
- Ezetimibe (Ezetrol)
- Gemfibrozil (Lopid)
- Nicotinic acid (Niacin)

Oxygen

- Administer oxygen and titrate as appropriate to assist in oxygenating myocardial tissue, especially in those hypoxic, in respiratory distress, or those at high risk.

Nitroglycerin

- Dilates the coronary arteries
- Increases blood flow to the damaged area of myocardium
- Dosage
  — 0.4 mg/tablet
  — 1 tablet sublingual every 5 min × 3 doses

Morphine Sulfate

- Analgesic
- ↓ Anxiety and tachypnea
- Relaxes bronchial smooth muscle
- Improves gas exchange

Thrombolytic Therapy

- Useful when infarction is diagnosed early and administered within protocol guidelines; there is a time imperative
- Streptokinase, alteplase, or tPA

- Administered IV
- Most effective if given within 6 hours of onset of chest pain
- Heparin therapy usually follows thrombolytic therapy.

Beta-Blockers
- Decrease heart rate
- Reduce workload of the heart
- Decrease oxygen demand of myocardium

Calcium Channel Blockers
- Decrease conduction through AV node
- Slow heart rate
- Decrease oxygen demand by myocardium

Medical Interventions
- Percutaneous transluminal coronary angioplasty (PTCA)
- Balloon angioplasty
- Intracoronary stents
- Coronary artery bypass graft (CABG)

Acute Myocardial Infarction (MI)
- Destruction of myocardial tissue due to lack of blood and oxygen supply
- Begins with occlusion of the coronary artery
- Ischemia, injury, infarction
- ST-elevation MI (STEMI) (traditional MI)
- Non-STEMI (common in women)

Ischemia
- Results from reduced blood flow and oxygen to the coronary arteries
- If not reversed, injury occurs.
- Ischemia lasting 20 minutes or longer is sufficient to produce irreversible tissue damage.
- ST depression on electrocardiogram (ECG)

Injury
- Prolonged interruption of oxygen supply and nutrients
- Cells still salvageable
- ST depression on ECG

Infarction
- Tissue necrosis and death
- Irreversible damage
- Scar tissue has no electrical stimulation or contractility.
- Within 24 hours of infarction, healing process begins.
- Pathological Q waves

Complications
- As many as 90% of clients suffer complications, including:
  — Dysrhythmias

— Cardiac failure
— Cardiogenic shock
— Thromboembolism
— Ventricular rupture

Signs and Symptoms

- Pain
  - Sudden onset; severity increases
  - May persist for hours or days; not relieved by rest or nitroglycerin
  - Heavy/constrictive
  - Located behind the sternum
  - May radiate to arms, back, neck, or jaw
- Cool, clammy skin
- Rapid, irregular, feeble pulse

Atypical Symptoms

- Women
  - Discomfort rather than pain
  - Shortness of breath
  - Extreme fatigue
- Client with diabetes
  - May be asymptomatic
  - Neuropathy
  - Dyspnea
- Elderly client
  - Confusion/delirium
  - Dizziness
  - Shortness of breath

Medical Diagnosis

- ECG (12 lead): ST-segment elevation, T-wave inversion, pathologic Q-wave formation
- Confirm by cardiac biomarkers
  - Creatine kinase (CK)-MB (CK2) 0% of total CK most specific but does not elevate for 24 hours
  - Myoglobin <90 mcg/L
  - Troponin T <0.20 ng/mL and troponin I <0.03 ng/mL

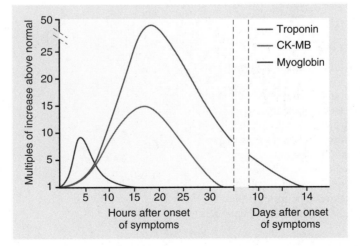

Figure 5-2 Serum cardiac markers found in the blood after myocardial infarction. (From Lewis, S., Dirksen, S., Heitkemper, M., & Bucher, L. (2014). *Medical-surgical nursing: Assessment and management of clinical problems* (9th ed.). St Louis: Mosby.)

Cardiac Lab Tests

- Troponin level
  - Troponins are found only in cardiac muscle.
  - May present as early after injury
  - Peaks within 24 hours
  - Returns to normal in 5 to 14 days
- Myoglobin level
  - Myoglobin is released 1 hour after an acute MI.
  - Rises before creatine kinase-MB levels
  - Returns to normal within 24 hours

Treatment

Overall goal is preserve myocardial tissue within 90 minutes of arrival to the healthcare facility with:

- Drug therapy
  - Oxygen
  - Nitroglycerin
  - Beta-blockers
  - Morphine
- Percutaneous coronary intervention (PCI) and stents
- Thrombolytic therapy via cardiac catheterization
- Standard of care is PCI within 90 minutes of presentation for medical care.
- If PCI is unavailable, then risk versus benefit ratio for thrombolytic therapy intravenously is completed.
- Coronary artery bypass graft
  - Used for severe CAD
  - Can be emergent or elective procedure
- Educate client on lowering modifiable risk factors

Heart Failure

Etiology

- CAD, prior MI
- Chronic HTN
- Cardiomyopathy
  - Dilated
  - Idiopathic
- Thyroid
- Diabetes
- Valvular and congenital heart disease
- Pulmonary diseases

Left-Sided Heart Failure (LHF)

- *Causes:* Left ventricular infarct, cardiomyopathy, hypertension
- *Symptoms:* Dyspnea, cough, orthopnea, pulmonary edema, paroxysmal nocturnal dyspnea
- *Signs:* S3 gallop, tachycardia, inspiratory rales beginning at lung bases, expiratory wheezes due to bronchospasms (misdiagnosed with asthma)
- *Laboratory findings:* ABGs reveal hypoxemia; chest radiograph shows pulmonary edema or pleural effusions, elevated b-type natriuretic peptide (BNP)
  - BNP levels greater than 500 ng/mL indicate heart failure is probable.

Right-Sided Heart Failure (RHF) Systemic Congestion

- *Causes:* LHF, RV infarct, pulmonary or tricuspid valve disease, pulmonary HTN, chronic obstructive pulmonary disease, PE
- *Symptoms:* Dyspnea on exertion, fatigue, weight gain, fluid retention
- *Signs:* Increased central venous pressure (CVP), jugular venous distention (JVD) >3 to 4 cm, hepatomegaly, ascites, peripheral or sacral edema; pleural and pericardial effusions are also not uncommon

Sodium and Volume Homeostasis

- As CO decreases, renal perfusion decreases.
- This activates the renin-angiotensin-aldosterone (RAAS) system.
- This causes fluid retention.

RHF Laboratory Tests

- Liver function shows hepatic congestion.
- Increased liver enzymes, increased prothrombin time, international normalized ratio
- Hyponatremia (fluid restriction only if Na^+ <132 mmol/L (mEq/L)
- Increased blood urea nitrogen/creatinine = decreased renal perfusion.

Pharmacological Management

- ACE inhibitors
  - Captopril
  - Enalapril sodium
  - Fosinopril sodium
  - Lisinopril
  - Quinapril hydrochloride
  - Ramipril
  - Perindopril erbumine
  - Benazepril hydrochloride
- Diuretics
  - Loop diuretics
    - Furosemide
    - Bumetanide
- Thiazides
  - Thiazide-related drug: hydrochlorothiazide
- Aldosterone antagonists
  - Spironolactone
- Inotropes
  - Digoxin
  - Dobutamine hydrochloride
- Phosphodiesterase inhibitors
  - Milrinone
- Natriuretic peptides
  - Nesiritide
- Beta-blockers
  - Metoprolol
  - Carvedilol
  - Bisoprolol
- Angiotensin II receptor blockers
  - Losartan potassium

- — Candesartan cilexetil
- — Valsartan
- ■ Vasodilators
  - — Nitrates: isosorbide dinitrate
  - — Hydralazine hydrochloride
  - — Sodium nitroprusside
  - — Prazosin hydrochloride
- ■ Dopamine agonist
  - — Dopamine hydrochloride
- ■ Analgesics
  - — Morphine sulfate
- ■ Anticoagulants
  - — Warfarin
- ■ Antiplatelet
- ■ Aspirin

Nursing and Collaborative Management

- ■ Administer oxygen as prescribed.
- ■ Repositioning and performing coughing and deep-breathing exercises every 2 hours
- ■ Diet
  - — Limit sodium intake.
  - — Fluid restriction only if Na^+ <132 mmol/L (mEq/L)
  - — Avoid excessive fluids.
  - — Avoid alcohol—depresses myocardial contractility
  - — With CAD: low cholesterol, low fat, low Na^+
- ■ Educate
  - — Signs of worsening condition such as weight gain (1.36 kg [3 lb] in a week or 0.454 to 0.9 kg [1 to 2 lb] overnight), increasing dyspnea on exertion, orthopnea, or paroxysmal nocturnal dyspnea
  - — Encourage regular exercise, which improves the function of skeletal muscle more than changes in myocardial function.

The nurse is administering 0900 medications to three clients on a telemetry unit when the UAP reports that another client is complaining of a sudden onset of substernal discomfort. What action should the nurse take?
A. Ask the UAP to obtain the client's vital signs.
B. Assess the client's discomfort.
C. Advise the client to rest in bed.
D. Observe the client's ECG pattern.

HESI Test Question Approach			
Positive?		YES	NO
Key Words			
Rephrase			
Rule Out Choices			
A	B	C	D

A 62-year-old client who has a history of coronary heart disease was admitted to the acute care unit 2 days ago for management of angina. During the assessment, the client states, "I feel like I have indigestion." In what order should the nurse implement care? (Arrange from first action to last.)

A. Notify the rapid response team.
B. Administer PRN (as needed) nitroglycerin prescription.
C. Check the pulse, respirations, blood pressure, and oxygen saturation.
D. Document assessment on the electronic medical record.
E. Provide 2 L of oxygen via nasal cannula.

HESI Test Question Approach

Positive?		YES	NO
Key Words			
Rephrase			
Rule Out Choices			
A	B	C	D	E

A client complains of a severe headache after receiving sublingual nitroglycerin 0.4 mg for angina. Which prescription should the nurse administer?

A. A second dose of nitroglycerin
B. A scheduled dose of low-dose aspirin
C. A PRN dose of acetaminophen PO
D. A PRN dose of morphine sulfate IV

HESI Test Question Approach

Positive?		YES	NO
Key Words			
Rephrase			
Rule Out Choices			
A	B	C	D

The nurse is caring for a client when the client suddenly becomes unconscious. The nurse identifies the following rhythm on the monitor. Which action is the highest priority?

A. Check for a carotid pulse.
B. Begin chest compressions.
C. Administer epinephrine 1:10,000 IV.
D. Initiate bag-valve mask ventilations.

HESI Test Question Approach

Positive?		YES	NO
Key Words			
Rephrase			
Rule Out Choices			
A	B	C	D

Dysrhythmias: Interpretation and Management

- Standard ECG (12 leads)
  — Provides best overall evaluation
- Telemetry
  — Usually three leads show one view of the heart.
- Holter monitor
  — Usually worn by client to obtain a 24-hour continuous reading

Electrocardiogram (ECG)

- P wave
  — Atrial depolarization
- QRS complex
  — Ventricular depolarization
  — Normal: <0.11 second
- ST segment
  — Early ventricular repolarization
- P-R interval
  — Reflects time required for impulse to travel through SA node
  — Normal: 0.12 to 0.20 second
- R-R interval
  — Reflects regularity of heartbeat

Dysrhythmias

- Client may be asymptomatic until cardiac output is altered.
- Client may complain of palpitations, syncope, pain, dyspnea, and diaphoresis.
- Changes seen in pulse rate/rhythm, as well as ECG changes
- Always treat the client, *not* the monitor.

Atrial Dysrhythmias

- A-fib (atrial fibrillation)
  — Chaotic activity in the AV node
  — No true P waves visible
  — Irregular R-R intervals
  — Risk for CVA
  — Anticoagulant therapy required
- Atrial flutter
  — Sawtoothed waveform
  — Regular R-R interval
  — Fluttering in the chest
  — Ventricular rhythm regular
- Cardioversion may be used to treat either type of atrial dysrhythmia.
- Collaborative care focuses on rate control.
- If onset is >48 hours, then a TEE is required.
- Always assure sedation prior to cardioversion.

Ventricular Dysrhythmias

- V-tach (ventricular tachycardia)
  — Wide, bizarre QRS complex
  — Assess whether client has a pulse.
  — Is the patient hemodynamically unstable? (Low blood pressure, diaphoresis, dizziness)
  — Prepare for synchronized cardioversion if a pulse is present.
  — Initiate basic and advanced life support guidelines if no pulse.
  — Administer antiarrhythmic drugs (amiodarone).
- V-fib (ventricular fibrillation)
  — Cardiac emergency
  — No cardiac output
  — Start cardiopulmonary resuscitation (CPR).
  — Defibrillate as quickly as possible.
  — Administer antiarrhythmic drugs.

Antiarrhythmic Medications

- **Class I:** sodium channel blockers (decrease conduction velocity in the atria, ventricles, and His-Purkinje system)
  - IA
    - Disopyramide
    - Procainamide hydrochloride (Procan SR)
    - Quinidine sulfate
  - IB
    - Lidocaine hydrochloride (Xylocaine)
    - Mexiletine hydrochloride
    - Phenytoin sodium (Dilantin)
  - IC
  - Flecainide acetate (Tambocor)
  - Propafenone hydrochloride (Rythmol)
  - Other Class I
    - Moricizine
- **Class II:** Beta-adrenergic blockers (decrease automaticity of the SA node, decrease conduction velocity in AV node)
  - Acebutolol hydrochloride (Rhotral, Sectral)
  - Atenolol (Tenormin)
  - Esmolol hydrochloride (Brevibloc)
  - Metoprolol tartrate (Lopressor)
  - Sotalol hydrochloride (Rylosol)
- **Class III:** potassium channel blockers (delay repolarization)
  - Amiodarone hydrochloride
  - Dofetilide (Tikosyn)
  - Sotalol hydrochloride (Betapace)
- **Class IV:** calcium channel blockers (decrease automaticity of SA node, delay AV node conduction)
  - Diltiazem hydrochloride (Cardizem)
  - Verapamil hydrochloride

Other Antidysrhythmic Drugs

- Adenosine (Adenocard)
- Digoxin (Lanoxin)
- Ibutilide fumarate (Corvert)
- Magnesium

A 60-year-old client who has a history of hypertension, heart failure, and sleep apnea is admitted to the acute care unit. Which finding(s) would relate most directly to a diagnosis of acute decompensated heart failure? (Select all that apply.)

A. Respiratory rate of 25 breaths/min
B. Orthopnea
C. S3 heart sound
D. Dry, nonproductive cough
E. Heart rate of 69 and irregular

HESI Test Question Approach			
Positive?		**YES**	**NO**
Key Words			
Rephrase			
Rule Out Choices			
A	B	C	D	E

Inflammatory Heart Disease

- Endocarditis
  - Signs/symptoms: fever, positive blood cultures, murmur, hemorrhages, heart failure symptoms, seen often with IV drug abuse
  - Infective endocarditis can lead to damaged heart valves.
  - Assess for right- or left-sided heart failure.
  - Administer IV antibiotics; therapy will continue for 4 to 6 weeks.
  - Maintain balance of rest and physical activity.
  - Surgical treatment if valvular damage occurs
  - Teach clients to request prophylactic antibiotics for every invasive procedure (dental included).
- Pericarditis
  - S/S: pain—hurts more with deep breath or supine, pericardial friction rub
  - Monitor for ST-segment elevation.
  - Monitor hemodynamic status.
  - Facilitate a leaning-over position and NSAIDs for pain control measures.

Valvular Heart Disease

- Valves may be unable to:
  - Fully open (stenosis)
  - Fully close (insufficiency or regurgitation)
- Causes
  - Rheumatic fever
  - Congenital heart disease
  - Syphilis
  - Endocarditis
  - Hypertension

Mitral Valve Stenosis

- Early period—may have no symptoms
- Later—excessive fatigue, dyspnea on exertion, orthopnea, dry cough, hemoptysis, or pulmonary edema
- Rumbling apical diastolic murmur and atrial fibrillation are common.

Nursing and Collaborative Management

See section on heart failure.
- Monitor for atrial fibrillation with thrombus formation.
- Give prophylactic antibiotic therapy before any invasive procedures (dental, surgical, childbirth).
- May require surgical repair or valve replacement
- With prosthetic valve replacement, teach client about need for lifelong anticoagulant therapy.

The nurse receives report on four clients on the cardiac unit. Which client should the nurse assess first?

A. The client with thrombophlebitis and a positive Homans sign
B. The client with left-sided heart failure and an S3 gallop
C. The client with pericarditis and inspiratory chest pain
D. The client with halo vision after digitalization

HESI Test Question Approach			
Positive?		**YES**	**NO**
Key Words			
Rephrase			
Rule Out Choices			
A	**B**	**C**	**D**

Vascular Disorders

Many individuals have arterial and venous disorders.

Arterial

- Smooth, shiny skin
- Pallor on elevation
- Weak or absent peripheral pulses
- Sharp or tingling pain
- Cool to touch
- Intermittent claudication (classic symptom)
- Painful, nonedematous ulcers
- Bruits

Venous

- Monitor for history of deep vein thrombosis.
- Bluish purple skin discoloration
- Normal peripheral pulses
- Warm to touch
- Slightly painful ulcers with marked edema

Nursing and Collaborative Management

General

- Change positions frequently; avoid sitting with crossed legs.
- Wear *no* restrictive clothing; do not cross legs.
- Maintain a warm environment; wear socks
- Avoid caffeine, nicotine, emotional stress.
- Keep extremities warm with clothing, not external heaters.
- Encourage smoking cessation.
- With thrombosis, administer thrombolytic agents and anticoagulants as ordered.

Arterial

- Bed rest
- Keep extremity below the level of the heart.
- Topical antibiotics
- Antiplatelets
- Surgical grafting intervention

Venous

- Wound care
- Diet that promotes wound healing: zinc and vitamins A and C

- Compression stockings day and evening
- Teach client to elevate legs (at least 20 minutes, 4 to 5 times/day)

Abdominal Aortic Aneurysm

- Pulsating abdominal mass, tearing chest, flank, or abdominal pain
- Bruit heard over abdomen
- Confirmed on radiograph
- With rupture: shortness of breath, hypovolemic shock (hypotension, diaphoresis, ↓ level of consciousness, oliguria)
- Postoperative care after surgical repair of aneurysm
  — Monitor for signs/symptoms of renal failure, myocardial infarction, acute respiratory distress syndrome, or postoperative ileus.
  — Changes in pulses, signs/symptoms of occluded graft (changes in pulses, pain, cyanotic extremities)

Venous Thromboembolism

- Inflammation of the venous wall with clot formation
- Signs/symptoms: calf pain, edema of calf, induration (hardening) along the blood vessel warmth and redness

NOTE: Pain in the calf on dorsiflexion of the foot (positive Homans sign) appears in only a small percentage of clients with DVT, and false-positive findings are common. Therefore, relying on a Homans sign is not advised.

- Restrict ambulation.
- Elevate extremity.
- Antiembolic stockings
- Refrain from massaging leg muscles.
- Medications
  — Heparin therapy
    • Therapeutic levels of aPTTs are usually 1.5 to 2 times normal control levels.
    • Protamine sulfate antidote
  — Coumadin therapy
    • Monitor prothrombin time (PT), international normalized ratio (INR).
    • Vitamin K: antidote
  — Antiplatelet agents
    • Ticlopidine (Ticlid)
    • Clopidogrel bisulfate (Plavix)

Which client should the nurse assess first?

A. The client receiving oxygen per nasal cannula who is dyspneic on mild exertion and has a hemoglobin of 70 mmol/L (7 g/dL)
B. The client receiving IV aminoglycosides per CVC who complains of nausea and has a trough level below therapeutic levels
C. The client receiving PRBCs who complains of flank pain and has a blood pressure of 98/52 mm Hg
D. The client receiving chemotherapy whose temperature is 37.2° C (98.9° F) and who has a WBC count of 2.5×10^9/L (2500/mm³)

HESI Test Question Approach		
Positive?	**YES**	**NO**
Key Words		
Rephrase		
Rule Out Choices		
A	**B**	**C**	**D**

Interpret the rhythm

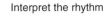

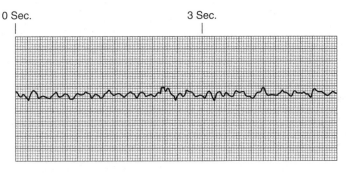

Ventricular Fibrillation. (From Urden L et al: *Critical care nursing: diagnosis and management*, ed 6, p 394, St. Louis, Mosby.)

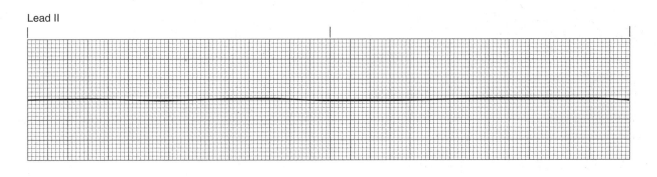

Asystole. (From Sole M, et al: *Introduction to critical care nursing*, ed. 6, p 128, Philadelphia, 2013, Saunders.)

6 Ingestion, Digestion, Absorption, and Elimination

The nurse is ordering afternoon snacks for several clients. Which client will benefit from a snack of cheese-and-bacon scrambled eggs with added protein powder?

A. The client with cirrhosis
B. The client with paralytic ileus
C. The client with cholelithiasis
D. The client with dumping syndrome

HESI Test Question Approach			
Positive?		**YES**	**NO**
Key Words			
Rephrase			
Rule Out Choices			
A	**B**	**C**	**D**

Gastroesophageal Reflux Disease (GERD)

- Not a disease but a syndrome
- Any clinically significant symptomatic condition secondary to reflux of gastric contents into the lower esophagus
- Most common upper gastrointestinal (GI) problem seen in adults

Etiology and Pathophysiology

There is no single cause of GERD. Predisposing conditions include:

- Incompetent lower esophageal sphincter (LES)
- Hiatal hernia
- Decreased esophageal clearance (ability to clear liquids or food from the esophagus into the stomach) resulting from impaired esophageal motility
- Decreased gastric emptying

Nursing Assessment

- Heartburn after eating
- Fullness and discomfort after eating
- Ask client what foods seem to aggravate symptoms
- Positive diagnosis from barium swallow or fluoroscopy (hiatal hernia)

Collaborative and Nursing Management

- Lifestyle modifications
- Encourage small, frequent meals.
- Sit up while eating and remain upright for 1 hour after eating.
- Stop eating 3 hours before bedtime.
- Elevate head of bed with 4- to 6-inch blocks.
- Take proton pump inhibitors to reduce production of acid from the stomach.
- H2-receptor antagonists to block the release of histamine 2, which produces acid

Peptic Ulcer Disease

- Significant gastric ulcers are caused by *Helicobacter pylori* bacteria.
- Risk factors
  - Drugs: nonsteroidal antiinflammatory drugs (NSAIDs), corticosteroids, aspirin
  - Alcohol, coffee
  - Cigarette smoking
  - Trauma
  - Stress

Nursing Assessment

- Left epigastric pain, may radiate to back
- Occurs 1 to 2 hours after meals
- Epigastric pain usually relieved with food
- Diagnosis
  - Barium swallow
  - Upper endoscopy

Collaborative and Nursing Management

- Onset of symptoms
- What relieves symptoms
- Monitor stools for bleeding.
- Administer antacids and antibiotics as ordered.
- Small, frequent meals are best.

Complications

- Uncontrolled bleeding or perforation
  - Prepare for immediate surgery
- Dumping syndrome—postoperative complication
  - Occurs 5 to 30 minutes after eating
  - Vertigo, syncope, tachycardia
  - Small, frequent meals
  - High-fat, high-protein, low-carbohydrate diet
  - Avoid liquids with meals

Client Teaching

- Avoid certain medications
  - Salicylates
  - NSAIDs
- Inform healthcare personnel of history of peptic ulcer disease.
- Symptoms of GI bleeding
  - Dark, tarry stools
  - Coffee ground emesis
  - Bright red rectal bleeding

Crohn's Disease (Regional Enteritis)

- Affects both small and large intestines
- Inflammation extends through all layers of intestine.
- Right lower quadrant abdominal pain
- Nausea and vomiting
- Three to four stools per day
- Barium enema shows narrowing with areas of stricture separated by segments of normal bowels.
- Capsule endoscopy has shown greater sensitivity than radiography for diagnosis.
- Fistulas can develop.

Nursing and Collaborative Management

■ Initial treatment is based on symptomatic relief, which usually includes parenteral replacement of fluids, electrolytes, and blood products. Complete bed rest and assistance with activities of daily living during acute phases are prescribed.

Pharmacotherapy

■ Sedatives and tranquilizers—to promote rest and reduce anxiety
■ Antidiarrheal medications—to reduce diarrhea and cramping
■ Sulfasalazine (Salazopyrin [Canada] Azulfidine, Azulfidine EN-tabs)—to treat acute exacerbations of colonic and ileocolonic disease
■ Corticosteroids (prednisone [Winpred])—to reduce the active inflammatory response
■ Immunosuppressive agents (infliximab [Remicade], adalimumab [Humira])—to allow dosage reduction or withdrawal of corticosteroids
■ Antimicrobials—to control infections and perianal fistulas

Nutritional Management

■ During acute exacerbations: total parenteral nutrition (TPN) and nothing by mouth (NPO; bowel rest)
■ Elemental diet
■ Bland diets
■ No milk, milk products
■ Supplementation of vitamins and minerals, especially calcium, iron, folate, magnesium, vitamin D

Surgical Management

■ Surgical management is reserved for complications rather than as a primary form of therapy. Common indications for surgery include bowel obstruction, internal and enterocutaneous fistulas, intraabdominal abscesses, and perianal disease.

Ulcerative Colitis

■ Occurs in the large bowel and rectum
■ Sigmoidoscopy and colonoscopy allow direct examination of the large intestinal mucosa and are used for diagnosis.
■ Symptoms
  — Bloody diarrhea
  — Abdominal pain
  — Liquid stools—10 to 20/day
  — Anemia

Nursing Interventions

■ Low-residue, low-fat, high-protein, high-calorie diet
■ No dairy products
■ Tepid fluids
■ Daily calorie count
■ Monitor intake and output (I & O)

- Medications
  - Corticosteroids
  - Antidiarrheals
  - Sulfasalazine (Salazopyrin [Canada], Azulfidine)
  - Infliximab (Remicade) or other biological treatments

Diverticular Diseases
- Left lower quadrant pain
- Signs and symptoms of intestinal obstruction
- Abdominal distention
- Constipation/diarrhea
- Positive barium enema
- Colonoscopy

Nursing and Collaborative Management
- High-fiber diet unless inflammation is present
- If inflammation is present:
  - NPO
  - Then low-residue, bland diet
  - Bulk-forming laxatives
  - Avoid heavy lifting, tight clothing, and straining.

Intestinal Obstruction
- Mechanical causes
  - Adhesions most common
  - Strangulated hernia
  - Tumors
- Neurogenic causes
  - Paralytic ileus
  - Spinal cord lesion
- Vascular cause
  - Mesenteric artery occlusion

Nursing Assessment
- Sudden abdominal pain
- History of obstruction
- High-pitched bowel sounds (early mechanical obstruction)
- Bowel sounds diminished or absent (neurogenic or late mechanical obstruction)

Nursing and Collaborative Management
- NPO
- Intravenous (IV) fluids
- Nasogastric tube to intermittent suction

Liver, Pancreas, and Biliary Tract Problems

A client is receiving pancreatic enzyme replacement therapy for chronic pancreatitis. Which statement by the client indicates a need for more effective teaching?
A. "I will need to mix the enzyme with a protein food."
B. "I will take the enzymes with each meal."
C. "My stools will decrease in number and frequency."
D. "My abdominal pain may lessen."

The nurse is providing discharge instructions to a client after a colon resection. Which statement by the client indicates that teaching has been effective?
A. "It is normal for the incision site to be warm."
B. "I will take my pain medications around the clock."
C. "I will call the healthcare provider if my temperature goes above 38° C (100.4° F)."
D. "I will resume sexual activity this week."

Cirrhosis
- Degeneration of the liver tissue
- Chronic progressive disease

Nursing Assessment
- Early sign: right upper quadrant pain
- History
  — Alcohol abuse
  — Street and prescription drug abuse
  — Exposure to hepatotoxins
  — Jaundice
- Dark-colored urine
- Clay-colored stools
- Yellow sclera
- Fruity or musty breath
- Asterixis
- Palmar erythema
- Ascites
- Weight loss

Esophageal Varices
- A common complication of cirrhosis; may rupture and cause hemorrhage

HESI Test Question Approach			
Positive?		YES	NO
Key Words			
Rephrase			
Rule Out Choices			
A	B	C	D

HESI Test Question Approach			
Positive?		YES	NO
Key Words			
Rephrase			
Rule Out Choices			
A	B	C	D

Treatment

- Esophagogastric balloon
- Vitamin K
- Blood products
- Coagulation factors

Nursing and Collaborative Management

- Monitor for bleeding.
  — Avoid injections.
  — Maintain pressure for 5 minutes after venipunctures.
- Provide skin care.
  — Avoid soap.
  — Apply lotions.
- Monitor fluid and electrolytes/ascites.
  — Accurate I & O.
  — Weigh daily.
  — Restrict fluids (1500 mL/day).
  — Abdominal girth
  — Prepare for paracentesis and peritoneovenous shunts.

Dietary Teaching

- May need to restrict protein
- Low sodium
- Low potassium
- Low fat
- High carbohydrate
- May need to take lactulose as ammonia detoxicant/stimulant laxative

Hepatitis

Widespread inflammation of liver cells, usually caused by a virus

Nursing Assessment

- Risk groups
  — Homosexual males
  — IV drug users (disease is transmitted by contaminated needles)
  — Tattoo/body piercing with contaminated needles
  — Those living in crowded conditions
  — Healthcare workers employed in high-risk areas
- Fatigue, weakness
- Anorexia, nausea
- Jaundice
- Dark urine
- Joint pain, muscle aches
- Elevated liver enzymes (alanine transaminase, aspartate transaminase, alkaline phosphatase), bilirubin

Nursing and Collaborative Management

- Frequent rest periods
- Provide high-calorie, high-carbohydrate diet with moderate fats and proteins.
- Administer antiemetic as needed.
- Limit alcohol intake and drugs detoxified by the liver.

Pancreatitis

- Acute: autodigestion of the pancreas
  — Alcohol ingestion and biliary tract disease are major causes.
- Chronic: progressive, destructive disease
  — Long-term alcohol use is a major factor in disease.

Acute Pancreatitis Assessment

Abdominal pain is the predominant symptom of acute pancreatitis.

- Located in the left upper quadrant
- Radiates to the back
- Sudden onset
- Described as severe, deep, piercing, and continuous
- Aggravated by eating and is not relieved by vomiting
- Accompanied by flushing, cyanosis, and dyspnea

Other Manifestations of Acute Pancreatitis

- Nausea and vomiting
- Low-grade fever
- Leukocytosis
- Jaundice
- Abdominal tenderness with muscle guarding
- Bowel sounds may be decreased or absent, and ileus may occur.
- Areas of ecchymoses, *Grey Turner's spots* or *sign,* a bluish flank discoloration and *Cullen's sign,* a bluish periumbilical discoloration
- Hypotension
- Tachycardia
- Hypovolemia (massive fluid shift into the retroperitoneal space)
- Shock (hemorrhage into the pancreas)
- Toxemia (activated pancreatic enzymes)
- Lungs frequently involved (crackles)

Chronic Pancreatitis Assessment

- Steatorrhea
- Diarrhea
- Jaundice
- Ascites
- Weight loss

Nursing and Collaborative Management

- Acute management
  — NPO
  — Nasogastric tube to suction
  — Morphine or hydromorphone are typically used for pain management.
  — Sitting up or leaning forward may reduce pain.
  — Monitor blood sugar.
  — Teach foods and fluids to avoid.
- Chronic management
  — Pain management
  — Morphine
  — Pancreatic enzymes
    • Mix powdered forms with fruit juice or applesauce; avoid mixing with proteins.
  — Histamine blocker agents
    • Teach foods and fluids to avoid.

A client who has an obstruction of the common bile duct caused by cholelithiasis passes clay-colored stools containing streaks of fat. What action should the nurse take?

A. Auscultate for diminished bowel sounds.
B. Send a stool specimen to the lab.
C. Document the assessment in the chart.
D. Notify the healthcare provider.

Cholecystitis and Cholelithiasis

- Cholecystitis: acute inflammation of the gallbladder
- Cholelithiasis: formation or presence of gallstones

Nursing Assessment

- Pain
- Fever
- Elevated white blood cells (WBCs)
- Abdominal tenderness
- Jaundice

Nursing Plans and Interventions

- Analgesics for pain
- NPO
- NG to suction
- IV antibiotics
- Low-fat diet
  — Avoid fried, spicy, and fatty foods.

Nursing and Collaborative Management

- Cholecystitis
  — IV hydration
  — Administer antibiotics
  — Pain management
- Cholelithiasis
  — Nonsurgical removal
    • Endoscopic retrograde cholangiopancreatography (ERCP)
    • Lithotripsy
  — Surgical approach
    • Cholecystectomy, laparoscopic or open

A client is admitted with gastric ulcer disease and GI bleeding. Which risk factor should the nurse identify in the client's history?

A. Eats heavily seasoned foods
B. Uses NSAIDs daily
C. Consumes alcohol every day
D. Follows an acid-ash diet

HESI Test Question Approach			
Positive?		YES	NO
Key Words			
Rephrase			
Rule Out Choices			
A	B	C	D

HESI Test Question Approach			
Positive?		YES	NO
Key Words			
Rephrase			
Rule Out Choices			
A	B	C	D

The nurse is caring for a client with peritonitis. Which information should the nurse report immediately to the healthcare provider?

A. Blood pressure readings of 92/64, 110/70, and 100/68 over the past hour
B. Urine output of 300 mL over the past 8 hours
C. Rebound tenderness and pain the client rates as a 7 on a 0 to 10 scale
D. Dry mucous membranes and nausea

HESI Test Question Approach			
Positive?		YES	NO
Key Words			
Rephrase			
Rule Out Choices			
A	B	C	D

Renal and Urological Problems

Urinary Tract Infections

- Obtain clean-catch midstream specimen.
- Administer antibiotics as ordered.
  - Take fully prescribed dose.
  - Do not skip doses.
- Encourage fluid intake of 3000 mL/day.
- Encourage voiding every 2 to 3 hours.
- Avoid tight clothing and bubble baths.

Urinary Tract Obstruction

- Caused by calculi or stones
- Location of pain can help locate stone.
  - Flank pain (stone usually in upper ureter)
  - Pain radiating to abdomen (stone likely in ureter or bladder)

Nursing and Collaborative Management

- Administer narcotics.
- Strain all urine for passing stones.
- Encourage high fluid intake.
  - 3 to 4 L/day
- Strict I & O
- May need surgical management

Benign Prostatic Hyperplasia

- Enlargement of the prostrate
  - Most common treatment: transurethral resection of the prostate (TURP)
  - Can be done with laser to burn out prostate
  - If prostate is too large, suprapubic approach is used.
- Assess for:
  - Increased urinary frequency/decreased output
  - Bladder distention (increases risk of spasm)

Nursing and Collaborative Management

- Preoperative teaching
  - Pain management
  - Oversized balloon catheter

- Bladder spasms
  — Common after surgery
  — Use antispasmodics
    • Belladonna and opium suppositories
    • Oxybutynin chloride (Ditropan)
    • Dicyclomine hydrochloride (Bentyl)
- Continuous bladder irrigation is typically done to remove blood clots and ensure drainage.
- Drainage should be reddish pink for 24 hours, clearing to light pink.
- Monitor color and amount of urine output.
- Notify physician if client has bright red bleeding with large clots.

Discharge Teaching
- Continue to drink 12 to 14 glasses of water per day.
- Avoid straining.
- Avoid strenuous activity, sports, lifting, and intercourse for 3 to 4 weeks.
- Report large amounts of blood or frank blood.

The charge nurse is making assignments on the renal unit. Which client should the nurse assign to a practical nurse who is new to the unit?
A. An older client who has thick, dark red drainage in a urinary catheter 1 day after a transurethral prostatic resection
B. A middle-aged client admitted with acute renal failure secondary to a reaction to IV pyelogram dye
C. An older client who has end-stage renal disease and complains of nausea after receiving digoxin
D. A middle-aged client who receives hemodialysis and has been prescribed epoetin alfa subcutaneous daily

A client is currently in the oliguric phase of acute kidney injury. Which finding(s) would the nurse expect to assess on the client? (Select all that apply.)
A. 450 mL urine output in 24 hours
B. Potassium of 6.2 mEq/L
C. Sodium (serum) 155 mEq/L
D. Metabolic alkalosis
E. Weight gain

HESI Test Question Approach			
Positive?		YES	NO
Key Words			
Rephrase			
Rule Out Choices			
A	B	C	D

HESI Test Question Approach				
Positive?			YES	NO
Key Words				
Rephrase				
Rule Out Choices				
A	B	C	D	E

Acute Kidney Injury

- A reversible syndrome if symptoms are caught early enough
- Remember:
  — Kidneys use 25% of normal cardiac output to maintain function.
  — Kidneys excrete 1 to 2 L of urine per 24 hours for adults.
  — Three types of acute renal failure (ARF)
    - Prerenal
    - Intrarenal
    - Postrenal

Prerenal Failure

- Etiological factors
  — Hemorrhage
  — Hypovolemia
  — Decreased cardiac output
  — Decreased renal perfusion

Intrarenal Failure

- Etiological factors
  — May develop secondary to prerenal failure
  — Nephrotoxins
  — Infections (glomerulonephritis)
  — Renal injury
  — Vascular lesions

Postrenal Failure

- Etiological factors for obstruction
  — Calculi
  — Benign prostatic hyperplasia (BPH)
  — Tumors
  — Strictures

Nursing Assessment

- Decreased urine output
- Weight gain
- Edema
- Diagnostic test results—oliguric phase
  — ↓ Urine output
  — ↑ Blood urea nitrogen (BUN) and creatinine
  — ↑ Potassium
  — ↓ Sodium (serum)
  — ↓ pH
  — Metabolic acidosis
  — ↑ Urine sodium
  — Fixed at 1.010 specific gravity
- Diagnostic test results—diuretic phase
  — ↑ Urine output
  — ↓ Fluid volume
  — ↓ Potassium
  — ↓ Sodium
  — ↓ Urine specific gravity
  — ↓ Urine sodium

Nursing and Collaborative Management

- Oliguric phase: give only enough fluids to replace losses + 400 to 500 mL/24 hr
- Strict I & O
- Monitor lab values closely.
- Watch for electrocardiogram changes.
- Monitor weight daily.

After hemodialysis, the nurse is evaluating the blood results for a client who has end-stage renal disease. Which value should the nurse verify with the laboratory?

A. Elevated serum potassium
B. Increase in serum calcium
C. Low hemoglobin
D. Reduction in serum sodium

HESI Test Question Approach			
Positive?		YES	NO
Key Words			
Rephrase			
Rule Out Choices			
A	**B**	**C**	**D**

Chronic Kidney Disease (CKD)

- End-stage renal disease
- Progressive irreversible damage to the nephrons and glomeruli
- Causes
  — Diabetic nephropathy
  — Hypertensive nephrosclerosis
  — Glomerulonephritis
  — Polycystic kidney disease

Nursing Assessment

- Early stage
  — Polyuria
  — Renal insufficiency
- Late stage
  — Oliguria
  — Hematuria
  — Proteinuria
  — Edema
  — Increased blood pressure
  — Muscle wasting secondary to negative nitrogen balance
  — Ammonia taste in mouth
  — ↑ Creatinine, ↑ phosphorus, ↑ potassium
- End stage
  — Anuria (<100 mL/24 hr)

Nursing and Collaborative Management

- Monitor serum electrolytes.
- Weigh daily.
- Strict I & O
- Renal diet
  — Low protein
  — Low sodium
  — Low potassium
  — Low phosphate

Medications

- Drugs are used to manage associated complications.
  — Aluminum hydroxide (to bind phosphates)
  — Epoetin (Eprex [Canada] Epogen) (to treat anemia)
  — Antihypertensive therapy
  — Calcium supplements and vitamin D
  — Antihyperlipidemics
  — Statins (to lower low-density lipoprotein cholesterol)
  — Fibrates (to lower triglycerides)
- CAUTION: As kidney function decreases, medication doses need adjustment.

Renal Dialysis

- Hemodialysis
  — AV fistula
- No venipunctures, IVs, or blood pressure taken in AV shunt arm
- Withhold medications that would affect hemodynamic stability before dialysis.
- Peritoneal dialysis
  — Monitor indwell and outflow times closely.
  — Monitor I & O.

Postoperative Care: Kidney Surgery

- Respiratory status
  — Auscultate to detect rales or rhonchi.
  — Demonstrate splinting method.
- Circulatory status
  — Monitor for shock.
  — Monitor surgical site for bleeding.
- Pain relief status
  — Administer narcotic analgesics as needed.
- Urinary status
  — Check urinary output and drainage from *all* tubes.
  — Strict I & O

A client with a 20-year history of type 1 diabetes mellitus is having renal function tests because of recent fatigue, weakness, BUN of 8.5 mmol/L (24 mg/dL), and a serum creatinine of 146 mcmol/L (1.6 mg/dL). What other early symptom of renal insufficiency might the nurse expect?

A. Dyspnea
B. Nocturia
C. Confusion
D. Stomatitis

HESI Test Question Approach			
Positive?		YES	NO
Key Words			
Rephrase			
Rule Out Choices			
A	B	C	D

A male client who has type 1 diabetes returns to the clinic for follow-up after dietary counseling. The client states that he has been managing his diabetes very closely. Which lab result indicates that the client is maintaining tight control of the disease?

A. Fasting blood sugar changes from 7.5 to 6 mmol/L (135 to 110 mg/dL)
B. Self-monitoring of blood glucose at bedtime changes from 2.5 to 5 mmol/L (45 to 90 mg/dL)
C. Glycosylated hemoglobin (hemoglobin $A1_C$) changes from 9% to 6%
D. Urine ketones change from 0 to 3

HESI Test Question Approach			
Positive?		YES	NO
Key Words			
Rephrase			
Rule Out Choices			
A	B	C	D

A 36-year-old married man with a body mass index (BMI) of 33 declares that he wants to lose weight. In addition to dietary intake and level of physical activity, what data are most necessary for the nurse to collect before planning care?

A. Draw blood for determination of a resting metabolic rate.
B. Determine who prepares the meals.
C. Identify the client's educational level.
D. Ascertain the client's smoking history.

HESI Test Question Approach			
Positive?		YES	NO
Key Words			
Rephrase			
Rule Out Choices			
A	B	C	D

Obesity, Metabolic Syndrome, Prediabetes, and Diabetes

■ **Primary obesity** develops when the calorie intake exceeds the body's metabolic needs.
■ Assessed by using a BMI chart
 — BMI of 18.5 to 24.9 kg/m^2: normal weight
 — BMI of 25 to 29.9 kg/m^2: overweight
 — BMI ≥30 kg/m^2: obese
 — BMI >40 kg/m^2: morbidly obese
■ Abdominal and visceral fat have been linked to metabolic syndrome.
■ Disproportionally represented in minority populations
■ Assessment
 — Risk-factor screening
  • Cardiovascular disease
  • Hypertension
  • Sleep apnea
  • Type 2 diabetes
  • Osteoporosis

Nursing and Collaborative Management

- Lifestyle management
  — Medical nutritional therapy
  — Physical activity
  — Behavior modification
- Pharmacological therapy
  — Orlistat: blocks fat breakdown in gastrointestinal (GI) tract
- Bariatric surgery
  — Criteria for bariatric surgery include a BMI ≥40 kg/m^2 or a BMI ≥35 kg/m^2 with one or more severe, obesity-related medical complications.
  — Gastric bypass, gastric banding, Roux-en-Y

Metabolic syndrome is a collection of risk factors that increase an individual's chance of developing cardiovascular disease and diabetes mellitus.

Assessment

- Meets three or more criteria:
  — **Waist circumference** ≥40 inches (102 cm) in men or ≥35 inches (88 cm) in women
  — **Triglycerides** >1.7 mmol/L (150 mg/dL) or drug treatment for elevated triglycerides
  — **High-density lipoprotein (HDL) cholesterol** <0.9 mmol/L (40 mg/dL in men or 1.1 mmol/L (<50 mg/dL in women) or drug treatment for reduced HDL cholesterol
  — **BP** ≥130 mm Hg systolic or ≥85 mm Hg diastolic or drug treatment for hypertension
  — **Fasting blood glucose level** ≥10 mmol/L (100 mg/dL) or drug treatment for elevated glucose

Nursing and Collaborative Management

- Lifestyle management
  — Medical nutritional therapy
  — Physical activity
  — Behavior modification

Prediabetes is a condition in which individuals are at increased risk for developing diabetes. In this condition, the blood glucose levels are high but not high enough to meet the diagnostic criteria for diabetes.

Assessment

- Fasting blood glucose level: 6.1 to 6.9 mmol/L (100 to 125 mg/dL)
- 2-hour oral glucose tolerance test (OGTT) values: 7.1 to 11 mmol/L (140 to 199 mg/dL)
- Glycosylated hemoglobin (hemoglobin A1$_C$): Canada —6.0% to 6.4%; United States—5.7% to 6.4%

Nursing and Collaborative Management

- Lifestyle management
  — Medical nutritional therapy
  — Physical activity
  — Behavior modification

Diabetes mellitus is a chronic multisystem disease related to abnormal insulin production, impaired insulin use, or both.

— *Type 1 diabetes:* Immune-mediated disease associated with absolute insulin deficiency. The body's own T cells destroy pancreatic beta cells, which are the source of insulin.

— *Type 2 diabetes:* The defect is insulin resistance and relative insulin deficiency. There is insufficient insulin production, insulin resistance, and/or excessive and unregulated glucose production from the liver.

— Other types of diabetes:
- Cystic fibrosis–related diabetes
- Transplant-related diabetes
- Gestational diabetes
- Steroid-induced diabetes
- Hospital-related hyperglycemia

Diagnosis

A1c%	Fasting Plasma Glucose	Oral Glucose Tolerance Test
≥6.5%	≥7.0 mmol/L (≥126 mg/dL)	≥11.1 mmol/L (≥200 mg/dL)

Clinical Manifestations

- Type 1
  - Abrupt onset of polyuria, polydipsia, polyphagia, and weight loss
  - Weakness and fatigue
  - Ketoacidosis may occur.
  - Serum glucose ≥14.0 mmol/L (250 mg/dL); ketonuria in large amounts
  - Arterial pH of <7.30 and Hco_3 <15 mmol/L (mEq/L)
  - Serum bicarbonate <15 mmol/L (mEq/dL), nausea, vomiting, dehydration, abdominal pain, Kussmaul's respirations, acetone odor to breath
  - Onset typically in childhood or adolescence but can occur at any age
- Type 2
  - Risk factors
    - Age >45 years
    - Overweight (BMI > 25)
    - First-degree relative with diabetes
    - Sedentary lifestyle
    - Ethnic at-risk group
    - Gestational diabetes or a baby >9 lb
    - Cardiovascular disease and/or hypertension
    - Abnormal lipids (low HDL, high triglycerides)
    - Previous impaired glucose or impaired fasting glucose test (prediabetes)
    - Polycystic ovarian syndrome
    - Signs of insulin resistance (acanthosis nigricans)
    - History of CV disease

- — Onset is insidious with polyuria, polyphagia, poly-dipsia, and weight loss; client may experience fatigue, recurrent infections, prolonged wound healing, blurred vision, and impotence.
- — Rare development of ketoacidosis; client is more likely to develop hyperosmolar hyperglycemia nonketotic syndrome (HHNKS) with blood sugars >33.3 mmol/L (600 mg/dL).
- — Plasma hyperosmolality
- — Dehydration
- — Altered mental status
- — Absent ketone bodies

Nursing Assessment

- Integument: skin breakdown
- Eyes: retinal problems, cataracts
- Kidneys: edema, urinary retention
- Periphery: cool skin, numbness, tingling
- Ulcerations on extremities and thick nails
- Cardiopulmonary angina and dyspnea

Nursing and Collaborative Management

- Medical nutrition therapy
  - — Type 1: integrate insulin with eating and exercise
  - — Type 2: heart-healthy diet and moderate weight loss of 10% to 20%
    - Space meals
    - Regular activity
- Monitoring
  - — Detects extremes and targets
  - — Educate client in techniques, calibration, and record keeping.
- Physical activity
  - — Moderate-intensity aerobic physical activity, 150 minutes per week; resistance training, 3 days per week
- Education
  - — Teach injection techniques.
  - — Refrigerate unopened insulin.
  - — Monitor for signs/symptoms of hypoglycemia.
  - — Foot care
  - — Manage sick days.
    - Keep taking insulin.
    - Check blood sugar more frequently.
    - Watch for signs/symptoms of hyperglycemia.

The registered nurse (RN) assigns the practical nurse (PN) a client with diabetes. Which findings should the RN instruct the PN to report immediately? Select all that apply.

A. Fingerstick blood sugar of 13.59 mmol/L (247 mg/dL)
B. Cold, clammy skin
C. Crackles at the end of inspiration
D. Numbness in the fingertips and toes
E. Unsteady gait, slurred speech

HESI Test Question Approach			
Positive?		**YES**	**NO**
Key Words			
Rephrase			
Rule Out Choices			
A	B	C	D	E

Pharmacological Intervention
Oral Agents and Injectables

- Key principles
  - Oral agents are not insulin; they work on the three defects of type 2 diabetes:
    - Insulin resistance
    - Decreased insulin production
    - Increased hepatic glucose production
- **Sulfonylureas:** increase insulin production from the pancreas; therefore, hypoglycemia is the major side effect.
  - Glipizide
  - Glyburide
  - Glimepiride
  - Gliclazide (Diamicron)
- **Meglitinides:** increase insulin production from the pancreas. They are short-acting and more rapidly absorbed and eliminated than sulfonylureas; therefore, hypoglycemia is a risk. Make sure client has a meal with each dose.
  - Repaglinide (GlucoNorm [Canada]; Prandin)
  - Nateglinide (Starlix)
- **Biguanides:** reduce glucose production by the liver and enhance insulin sensitivity at the tissue level. These are the first-choice drugs for most people with type 2 diabetes. Do not use in clients with kidney disease, liver disease, or heart failure or for clients who drink excessive amounts of alcohol.
  - Metformin hydrochloride
- **Alpha-glucosidase inhibitors** (starch blockers): slow the absorption of carbohydrate in the small intestine. Flatus is a common side effect.
  - Acarbose
- **Thiazolidinediones** (insulin sensitizers): most effective for clients with insulin resistance; do not cause hypoglycemia when used alone
  - Pioglitazone hydrochloride (Actos)
  - Rosiglitazone maleate (Avandia)
  - Do not use thiazolidinediones in clients with heart failure because of increased risk of myocardial infarction and stroke.
- **Dipeptidyl peptidase-4 (DPP-4) inhibitor:** inhibits DPP-4, thus slowing the inactivation of incretin hormones. Because the DPP-4 inhibitors are glucose dependent, they lower the potential for hypoglycemia.
  - Sitagliptin phosphate (Januvia)
  - Saxagliptin hydrochloride (Onglyza)
- **Incretin mimetic:** simulate one of the incretin hormones found to be decreased in people with type 2 diabetes. A prefilled pen is used to administer the drug subcutaneously. Acute pancreatitis and kidney problems have been associated with the use of these drugs.

Insulin Pharmacokinetics After Subcutaneous Injection

- Rapid-acting insulin: can be given IV
  - Glulisine (Apidra)—given within 15 minutes of meal
    - Onset: 0.25 hour

- Peak: 1 hour
- Duration: 2 to 3 hours
  — Lispro (Humalog)—given within 15 minutes of meal
  - Onset: 0.25 hour
  - Peak: 1 hour
  - Duration: 4 hours
  — Aspart (NovoRapid [Canada]; NovoLog)—given within 15 minutes of meal
  - Onset: 0.5 hour
  - Peak: 1 to 3 hours
  - Duration: 3 to 5 hours
  — Regular (Humulin R)—given within 30 minutes of meal
  - Onset: 0.5 to 1 hour
  - Peak: 2 to 4 hours
  - Duration: 5 to 7 hours
- **Intermediate-acting insulin:** do not give IV; can be mixed with rapid-acting insulins (see "Combinations" section).
  — Insulin isophane suspension (Humulin N)
  - Onset: 1 to 2 hours
  - Peak: 4 to 12 hours
  - Duration: 16 to 24 hours
- **Long-acting insulin:** cannot be mixed with any other type of insulin. Usually given once a day in the morning. Acts as basal insulin. Do not shake solutions. CAUTION: Solution is clear; do not confuse with regular insulin.
  — Glargine (Lantus)
  - Onset: 1 to 5 hours
  - Peak: Plateau
  - Duration: 24 hours
  — Detemir (Levemir)
  - Onset: 3 to 4 hours
  - Peak: Peakless
  - Duration: 24 hours

Combinations (Premix Insulins)
- Regular insulin 30% and Insulin Isophane (Humulin N) 70% (Canada): Humulin 30/70 (Canada); NPH and Regular (70% NPH insulin and 30% regular insulin):
  — Onset: 0.5 to 1 hour
  — Peak: 1.5 to 12 hours
  — Duration: Up to 24 hours
- Lispro insulins: Insulin Lispro protamine suspension 75% and insulin lispro 25% (Humalog Mix 25) (Canada); 75/25 (75% insulin lispro protamine suspension and 25% insulin lispro)
  — Onset: 0.25 to 0.5 hour
  — Peak: ≥2 hours
  — Duration: approximately 22 hours
  — Lispro: Lispro protamine suspension 50% and insulin lispro 50% (Humalog Mix 50) (Canada); protamine suspension 50% and insulin lispro 50% (Humalog Mix 50): 50/50 (50% insulin lispro protamine suspension and 50% insulin lispro)
  — Onset: 0.25 to 0.5 hour
  — Peak: 0.5 to 1.5 hours
  — Duration: approximately 22 hours

- Aspart insulins: 30% soluble insulin aspart and 70% insulin aspart protamine crystals (NovoMix 30) (Canada); 70/30 (70% insulin aspart protamine suspension and 30% insulin aspart)
  — Onset: 0.17 to 0.33 hour
  — Peak: 1 to 4 hours
  — Duration: Up to 24 hours
- Because analog premixed insulin has a rapid onset, it should be given shortly before meals and should not be given at bedtime. Clients who choose to use premixed insulin preparations should have a fairly routine lifestyle.
- In clients with impaired liver or kidney function, the insulin dosage may need to be reduced because insulin is metabolized by the liver and excreted by the kidneys.

The nurse is reviewing the current medication list of a client newly diagnosed with type 1 diabetes who will be prescribed insulin. Which medications should the RN discuss with the physician? (Select all that apply.)
A. Prednisone
B. Atenolol
C. Clarithromycin
D. Acetaminophen
E. Ibuprofen
F. Pantoprazole sodium

HESI Test Question Approach					
Positive?				**YES**	**NO**
Key Words					
Rephrase					
Rule Out Choices					
A	B	C	D	E	F

A client who was recently prescribed metformin hydrochloride calls the clinic to discuss symptoms of bloating, nausea, cramping, and diarrhea. Which instructions should the nurse provide the client? (Select all that apply.)
A. Discontinue the medication immediately.
B. Increase fiber and fluids in the diet.
C. Monitor the symptoms.
D. Continue to take the metformin as prescribed.
E. Seek immediate emergency medical care.

HESI Test Question Approach					
Positive?				**YES**	**NO**
Key Words					
Rephrase					
Rule Out Choices					
A	B	C	D	E	

Other Endocrine Problems

Which clinical manifestations would the nurse expect to assess in a client experiencing Graves disease? (Select all that apply.)

A. Tachycardia
B. Decreased sweating
C. Insomnia
D. Increased respiratory rate
E. Muscular aches and pains

HESI Test Question Approach			
Positive?		**YES**	**NO**
Key Words			
Rephrase			
Rule Out Choices			
A	B	C	D	E

Which client should the nurse assess first?

A. The client with hyperthyroidism exhibiting exophthalmos
B. The client with type 1 diabetes with an inflamed foot ulcer
C. The client with Cushing's syndrome exhibiting moon facies
D. The client with Addison's disease showing tremors and diaphoresis

HESI Test Question Approach			
Positive?		**YES**	**NO**
Key Words			
Rephrase			
Rule Out Choices			
A	B	C	D

Thyroid Gland Feedback Loop

Hypothalamus

⇩

TRH (+)
Anterior pituitary
— T_3 and T_4 (−) TSH (+)
— Thyroid gland

Hyperthyroidism

Nursing Assessment

- Enlarged thyroid gland
- Exophthalmos
- Weight loss
- T_3 elevated
- T_4 elevated
- Diarrhea
- Tachycardia
- Bruit over thyroid

Nursing Plans and Interventions

- Diet: high protein, high calorie, low caffeine, low fiber
- Treatment may trigger hypothyroidism; client may need hormone replacement.
- Propylthiouracil (PTU) therapy to block the synthesis of T_3 and T_4

- Iodine (^{131}I), a radioactive therapy to destroy thyroid cells
- Surgical management
  — Thyroidectomy
    - Position in high Fowler's.
    - Check behind neck for drainage.
    - Support neck when moving client.
    - Avoid flexion of the neck.
    - Assess for laryngeal edema.
    - Have tracheotomy set, oxygen, and suction equipment at bedside.
    - Have calcium gluconate or gluceptate at bedside.

Which adaptation of the environment is most important for the nurse to include in the plan of care for a client with myxedema?
A. Reduce environmental stimuli.
B. Prevent direct sunlight from entering the room.
C. Maintain a warm room temperature.
D. Minimize exposure to visitors.

HESI Test Question Approach		
Positive?	**YES**	**NO**
Key Words		
Rephrase		
Rule Out Choices		
A	B	C	D

Hypothyroidism

- Fatigue
- Bradycardia
- Weight gain
- Constipation
- Periorbital edema
- Cold intolerance
- Low T_3 (<70 ng/dL)
- Low T_4 (<5 ng/dL)

Nursing Plans and Interventions

- Myxedema coma (acute exacerbation of hypothyroidism): maintain airway
- Teach medication regimen.
- Monitor for side effects of medications.
- Monitor bowel program for signs/symptoms of constipation.

Medications

- **Levothyroxine** sodium (Eltroxin, Euthyrox, Synthroid)
  — Take first thing in AM before eating.
  — Monitor heart rate.
  — Hold for pulse >100 beats/min.
- Liothyronine (Cytomel)
  — Increases metabolic rate
  — Acts as synthetic T_3
  — Check hormone levels regularly.
  — Avoid food containing iodine.
- **Levothyroxine** (T_4) + liothyronine (T_3) (Liotrix)
  — Rapid onset

The nurse suspects a postoperative thyroidectomy client may have had the inadvertent removal of the parathyroid when the client begins to experience which symptoms? (Select all that apply.)

A. Hematoma formation
B. Harsh, vibratory sounds on inspiration
C. Tingling of lips, hands, and toes
D. Positive Chvostek's sign
E. Sensation of fullness at the incision site

HESI Test Question Approach

Positive?		YES	NO
Key Words			
Rephrase			
Rule Out Choices			

A	B	C	D	E

A client is admitted to the hospital with a diagnosis of Addison's crisis. The nurse places a peripheral saline lock. Regarding which prescription(s) should the nurse question the healthcare provider? (Select all that apply.)

A. IV D5NS at 300 mL/hr for 3 hours
B. Hydrocortisone sodium succinate 100 mg IV push
C. Potassium 20 mEq in 100 mL saline IV over 60 minutes
D. 50% dextrose intravenous push
E. 10% calcium chloride 5 mL intravenously over 10 minutes

HESI Test Question Approach

Positive?		YES	NO
Key Words			
Rephrase			
Rule Out Choices			

A	B	C	D	E

Addison's Disease

Etiology

- Sudden withdrawal from corticosteroids
- Hyposecretion of adrenal cortex hormones
- Lack of pituitary ACTH

Signs and Symptoms

- Progressive weakness
- Weight loss
- Nausea/vomiting
- Hypovolemia
- Hypoglycemia
- Hyponatremia
- Hyperkalemia
- Loss of body hair
- Postural hypotension
- Hyperpigmentation

Nursing Plans and Interventions

- Frequent vital signs
- Weigh daily
- Monitor fluid balance and serum electrolytes.
- Monitor for muscle weakness.
- Monitor serum glucose levels.
- Diet: high sodium, low potassium, high carbohydrates

- Encourage at least 3 L of fluid per day.
- Wear medic alert bracelet.
- Monitor for symptoms of overdosage/underdosage of corticosteroid and mineralocorticoid therapy.
- Carry emergency kit with 100 mg intramuscular corticosteroid.

Cushing's Syndrome and Cushing's Disease

Cushing's syndrome: excess adrenocorticoid activity caused by adrenal, pituitary, or hypothalamus tumors. Most common cause is iatrogenic administration of exogenous corticosteroids

Cushing's disease: excess adrenorticoid activity due to an adrenocorticotropic hormone—secreting pituitary adenoma

Nursing Assessment

- Moon face and edema of lower extremities
- Flat affect, irritability, anxiety, depression, psychosis
- Truncal obesity
- Abdominal striae
- Buffalo hump (fat deposits)
- Muscle atrophy, weakness
- Thin dry pale skin
- Hypertension
- Osteoporosis
- Immunosuppressed
- Hirsutism
- Lab results
  — Hyperglycemia
  — Hypernatremia
  — Hypocalcemia
  — Hypokalemia
  — Increased plasma cortisol levels

Nursing Plans and Interventions

- Monitor for signs/symptoms of infection
- Fever
- Skin lesions
- Elevated white blood cell count
- Wear medic alert bracelet
- Avoid extreme temperatures, infections, emotional disturbances
- Diet
  — Low sodium
  — Low carbohydrate

Sexually Transmitted Diseases (STDs)

- Symptoms and treatment vary by disease.
- Teach safer sex.
  — Limit number of partners.
  — Abstinence, mutual monogamy
  — Use latex condoms.
  — Lifestyle risks: drugs and alcohol
- Report incidence of STDs to appropriate health agencies.

Refer to review manuals for more in-depth information about STDs:

- *Evolve Reach Comprehensive Review for the NCLEX-RN Examination* (powered by HESI)
- *Mosby's Comprehensive Review of Nursing for the NCLEX-RN Examination*
- *Saunders Comprehensive Review for the NCLEX-RN Examination*

Female Reproductive Problems

A 52-year-old client who had an abdominal hysterectomy for cervical adenocarcinoma in situ is preparing for discharge. Which recommendation about women's health and screening examinations should the nurse offer?
A. Continue the annual Pap smear and mammogram, biannual clinical breast examinations, and monthly breast self-examinations (BSE).
B. A Pap smear is no longer necessary, but continue the annual mammogram and biannual clinical breast examinations, plus monthly BSE.
C. If the ovaries have been removed, only an annual mammogram and clinical breast examinations are necessary.
D. Annual mammograms are not needed if biannual clinical breast examinations and weekly BSE are done.

HESI Test Question Approach			
Positive?		YES	NO
Key Words			
Rephrase			
Rule Out Choices			
A	B	C	D

Benign Uterine Tumors
- Arise from muscle tissue of the uterus
- Signs and symptoms
  — Menorrhagia
  — Uterine enlargement
  — Dysmenorrhea
  — Anemia secondary to menorrhagia
  — Uterine enlargement
  — Low back pain and pelvic pain
  — Tend to disappear after menopause
- Nonsurgical options
  — Magnetic resonance—guided focused ultrasound
- Surgical options
  — Myomectomy
  — Hysterectomy
  — Fertility issues

After stopping hormone replacement therapy (HRT), a 76-year-old client reports she is experiencing increased vaginal discomfort during intercourse. What action should the nurse take?
A. Suggest the use of a vaginal cream or lubricant.
B. Recommend that the client abstain from sexual intercourse.
C. Teach the client to perform Kegel exercises daily.
D. Instruct the client to resume HRT.

HESI Test Question Approach			
Positive?		YES	NO
Key Words			
Rephrase			
Rule Out Choices			
A	B	C	D

Pelvic Organ Prolapse (POP): Uterine Prolapse, Cystocele, and Rectocele

- Preventive measures
  - Postpartum perineal exercises (Kegel)
  - Spaced pregnancy
  - Weight control
- Differing signs/symptoms for each condition
- Surgical intervention
  - Hysterectomy
  - Anterior and posterior vaginal repair
- Pain management postoperative
- Monitor urinary output postoperative.
- Observe for signs/symptoms of postoperative bleeding and infection.

A client who had a vaginal hysterectomy the previous day is saturating perineal pads with blood and requires frequent changes during the night. What is the nurse's priority action?

A. Provide iron-rich foods on each dietary tray.
B. Monitor the client's vital signs every 2 hours.
C. Administer IV fluids at the prescribed rate.
D. Encourage postoperative leg exercises.

HESI Test Question Approach			
Positive?		YES	NO
Key Words			
Rephrase			
Rule Out Choices			
A	B	C	D

The nurse assigned to the women's health unit received the morning report. Which client should the nurse assess first?

A. A 49-year-old client 1 day post vaginal hysterectomy who is saturating pads every 3 hours
B. A 34-year-old client post uterine artery embolization whose indwelling catheter was removed 4 hours ago and has not voided
C. A 52-year-old client 2 days post abdominal hysterectomy requesting oral analgesics instead of the PCA pump
D. A 67-year-old client 1 day post anterior and posterior repair who is refusing to ambulate with the UAP

HESI Test Question Approach			
Positive?		YES	NO
Key Words			
Rephrase			
Rule Out Choices			
A	B	C	D

Male Reproductive Problems

Etiology and Pathophysiology

Prostatitis is one of the most common male urologic disorders.

Common Manifestations (Acute Bacterial Prostatitis)

- Fever
- Chills
- Back pain

- Perineal pain
- Dysuria
- Urinary frequency
- Urgency
- Cloudy urine

Diagnostic Studies
- Urinalysis (UA)
- Urine culture
- White blood cell (WBC) count
- Blood cultures
- Prostate-specific antigen test (may be done to rule out prostate cancer)

Management
- Antibiotics
  — Sulfamethoxazole—trimethoprim (cotrimoxazole [Canada])
  — Ciprofloxacin hydrochloride
  — Ofloxacin (Apo-Ofloxacin [Canada])
  — Doxycycline hyclate
  — Tetracycline
- Antiinflammatory agents for pain control

Nursing Intervention
- Encourage fluid intake

Sexual Functioning
- **Vasectomy:** Bilateral surgical ligation of the vas deferens performed for the purpose of sterilization
- **Erectile dysfunction (ED):** Inability to attain or maintain an erect penis. ED can result from a large number of factors. Causes can include:
  — Diabetes
  — Vascular disease (the most common cause)
  — Side effects from medications
  — Result of surgery (prostatectomy)
  — Trauma
  — Chronic illness
  — Decreased gonadal hormone secretion
  — Stress
  — Difficulty in a relationship
  — Depression
  — Drugs and alcohol

The treatment for ED is based on the underlying cause.

Oral Drug Therapy
- Sildenafil citrate
  — Dosage: 25 to 100 mg by mouth, one dose per day, 1 hour before sexual activity
- Tadalafil
- Vardenafil hydrochloride
  — These drugs may potentiate the hypotensive effect of nitrates; they are contraindicated for individuals taking nitrates (e.g., nitroglycerin).
  — Teach to seek medical attention for an erection lasting longer than 4 hours (priapism).
  — Use with caution in elderly because drugs are slow to metabolize and be excreted.

8 Movement, Coordination, and Sensory Input

Altered State of Consciousness

- Glasgow Coma Scale
  — Used to assess level of consciousness
  — Maximum score 15, minimum 3
  — Score ≤7 = Coma
  — Score 3 to 4 = High mortality rate
  — Score >8 = Good prognosis
- Neurological vital signs
  — Pupil size (with sizing scale)
  — Limb movement (with scale)
  — Vital signs (blood pressure, temperature, pulse, respirations)

Table 8-1 Glasgow Coma Scale*

Variable	Response	Score
Eye opening	Spontaneously	4
	To verbal command	3
	To pain	2
	No response	1
Motor response	To verbal command	6
	Localizes pain	5
	Flexes/withdraws	4
	Flexor posturing (decorticate)	3
	Extensor posturing (decerebrate)	2
	No response	1
Verbal response	Oriented and converses	5
	Confused conversation	4
	Inappropriate words	3
	Incomprehensible sounds	2
	None	1

*The highest possible score is 15.
Ignatavicius, W. *Medical-Surgical Nursing: Patient-Centered Collaborative Care, 7th edition.* W. B. Saunders Company, 2013.

Nursing Assessment

- Assess for early signs/symptoms of changes in level of consciousness (LOC), which is the most sensitive and reliable indicator.
  — Decreasing LOC
  — Change in orientation
- Late signs
  — Cushing's triad
    • Widening pulse pressure
    • Slowing heart rate with full bounding pulse
    • Slowing and irregular respirations
  — Change in size, response of pupils, dilated on side of injury initially
  — Elevated temperature
- Assess for change in respiratory status.
  — Cheyne-Stokes respiration

- Maintain airway—with decreasing LOC will need mechanical ventilation
- Prevent hypoxia
  — Hyperventilate before suctioning
  — Limit suctioning to 15 seconds
    - Keep airway free of secretions
    - Position head to side

Treatment: Increased Intracranial Pressure (ICP)

- ICP monitoring
  — Goal ICP: <20 mm Hg
  — Hyperosmotic agents 20% mannitol
  — Steroids (use associated with increased risk of infections)
    - Dexamethasone (Decadron)
    - Methylprednisolone (Solu-Medrol)
- Barbiturates
- Prophylactic: Phenytoin sodium (Dilantin)
- Diuretics
  — Alternate with mannitol.
  — Avoid narcotics!
- Controlled hyperventilation
- Mild hypothermia
- Cerebrospinal fluid (CSF) drainage
  — Infection is a serious complication and systemic antibiotics are often ordered prophylactically.

Which change in the status of a client being treated for increased intracranial pressure warrants immediate action by the nurse?
A. Urinary output changes from 20 to 50 mL/hr
B. Arterial P_{CO_2} changes from 40 to 30 mm Hg
C. Glasgow Coma Scale score changes from 5 to 7
D. Pulse changes from 88 to 68 beats/min

HESI Test Question Approach			
Positive?		**YES**	**NO**
Key Words			
Rephrase			
Rule Out Choices			
A	**B**	**C**	**D**

Head Injury
Assessment

- Changes in LOC (i.e., confusion, combativeness)
- Signs of increased ICP
- Changes in vital signs
- Headache
- Vomiting
- Pupillary changes
- Seizure
- Ataxia
- Extremity motor strength and use—reflexes depressed or hyperactive
- Abnormal posturing (decerebrate or decorticate)

CSF Leakage

- Risk for meningitis with leakage
- May not see usual signs of increased ICP with leakage of CSF

- Drainage may come from nose (rhinorrhea) or ears (otorrhea).
- Altered cerebral perfusion related to ↑ ICP
  — MAP − ICP = CPP
  — Amount of blood flow from systemic circulation required to provide oxygen to the brain
  — Ideally cerebral perfusion pressure (CPP) should be >70 mm Hg.

Nursing Interventions
- Neurological assessment every 15 minutes
- Notify health care provider at *first* sign of deterioration.
- Limit visitors.
- Keep room quiet.
- Prevent straining.
- Keep HOB at 30 to 45 degrees.
- Avoid neck flexion/straining.
- Monitor intake and output (I & O).

The nurse is planning a class on stroke prevention for clients with hypertension. What information is most important to provide to the class?
A. Salt restriction diet
B. Weight reduction
C. Medication compliance
D. Risk for stroke

HESI Test Question Approach			
Positive?		**YES**	**NO**
Key Words			
Rephrase			
Rule Out Choices			
A	B	C	D

During the evaluation, which assessments indicate an early sign of increased ICP for a client newly diagnosed with a cerebral vascular accident? Select all that apply.
A. Alteration in the ability to respond to questions
B. Alteration in the ability to respond to verbal stimuli
C. Consensual response of pupils
D. Heart rate 50, blood pressure 192/60
E. Drooping of the mouth on one side

HESI Test Question Approach				
Positive?			**YES**	**NO**
Key Words				
Rephrase				
Rule Out Choices				
A	B	C	D	E

Stroke (Brain Attack) or Cerebrovascular Accident
- **Stroke** is a sudden loss of brain function caused by a disruption in the blood supply to part of the brain. Strokes are classified as ischemic or hemorrhagic.
  — *Ischemic stroke:* A clot may be thromboembolic or embolic, causing minimal or absent blood flow to the neurons.
  — *Hemorrhagic stroke:* May be a subarachnoid hemorrhage (SAH; bleeding into the subarachnoid

space) or an intracranial hemorrhage (direct bleeding into the brain tissue).

- **Transient ischemic attack (TIA):** A transient episode of neurological dysfunction caused by focal brain, spinal cord, or retinal ischemia, but without acute infarction of the brain. Clinical symptoms typically last less than 1 hour. Most fully resolve.

Assessment

- Risk factors
  - Cardiovascular disease (CVD), hypertension, previous TIA
  - Diabetes
  - Advanced age
  - History of atrial fibrillation or flutter
  - Oral contraceptives and hormone replacement therapy
  - Smoking
  - Alcohol: >2 drinks/day

The presenting symptoms relate to the specific area of the brain that has been damaged.

- Motor loss—hemiparesis or hemiplegia
- Communication loss—dysarthria, dysphasia, aphasia, or apraxia
- Perceptual disturbance—visual, spatial, and sensory
- Impaired mental acuity or psychological loss—decreased attention span, memory loss, depression, lability, hostility
- Bladder dysfunction may be either incontinence or retention
- Face, arms, speech, time (FAST)

Nursing and Collaborative Management

- IV tissue plasminogen activator (tPA) improves the neurological outcome in clients with stroke, who meet fibrinolytic criteria, when administered within 3–4.5 hours of onset. The client must be screened for intracranial bleeding before administration.
- Rehabilitation starts as soon as the client is stable.
- Mobility
- Speech
- Activities of daily living (ADLs)
- Elimination

The nurse is planning a class on stroke prevention for clients with hypertension. What information reflects accurate prevention measures that the clients can undertake?
A. Limit salt intake to 1500 mg/day or less.
B. Eliminate tobacco products.
C. Initiate a program of walking 1 mile per day.
D. Achieve a body mass index (BMI) of 26.2.
E. Schedule routine health assessments biannually.

HESI Test Question Approach			
Positive?		YES	NO
Key Words			
Rephrase			
Rule Out Choices			
A	B	C	D	E

Which client should be assigned to a graduate nurse being oriented to the neurological unit?

A. A client with a head injury who has a Glasgow Coma Scale score of 6
B. A client who developed autonomic dysreflexia after a T6 spinal cord injury
C. A client with multiple sclerosis who needs the first dose of interferon
D. A client suspected of having Guillain-Barré syndrome

The nurse is providing dietary education to a patient who is receiving levodopa. The nurse knows that education has been effective when the patient selects which safe meal choices? (Select all that apply.)

A. Scrambled eggs, two sausage patties, and skim milk
B. Oatmeal and orange juice
C. Whole wheat toast and tuna salad.
D. Spinach salad with avocados and sunflower seeds
E. Peanut butter and jelly sandwich, apple sauce, almond milk

Parkinson's Disease

- Chronic, progressive, debilitating neurological disease
- Triad of symptoms
  — Rigidity
    • Masklike face
    • Akinesia
    • Difficulty initiating and continuing movement
  — Bradykinesia
  — Tremors
    • Resting tremors
    • Pill rolling

Nursing and Collaborative Management

- *Safety* is always a priority!
- Take medications with meals.
- Change positions slowly to reduce postural hypotension.
- Thicken liquids.
- Soft foods
- Encourage activity and exercise.

Drug Therapy

- Dopaminergics
  — Levodopa (L-dopa, dopamine)
  — Blocks breakdown of levodopa to allow more levodopa to cross the blood-brain barrier
  — Avoid foods high in vitamin B_6 and high-protein foods
  — Levodopa-carbidopa (Sinemet, Parcopa [orally dissolving tablet])
  — Allows for less use of levodopa and helps decrease side effects

HESI Test Question Approach			
Positive?		YES	NO
Key Words			
Rephrase			
Rule Out Choices			
A	B	C	D

HESI Test Question Approach				
Positive?			YES	NO
Key Words				
Rephrase				
Rule Out Choices				
A	B	C	D	E

- Dopaminergic agonists
  — Bromocriptine mesylate (Parlodel)
    • Helps with motor fluctuations
  — Pramipexole (Mirapex)
  — Ropinirole hydrochloride (Requip)
  — Amantadine (Symmetrel)
- Anticholinergics—treat tremors
  — Trihexyphenidyl (Trihexyphen [Canada]; Artane)
  — Benztropine mesylate (Cogentin)
  — Procyclidine hydrochloride (Akineton)
- Antihistamine
  — Diphenhydramine (Benadryl)
- Monoamine oxidase inhibitors
  — Selegiline hydrochloride (Anipril [Canada]; Eldepryl)
- Catechol-*O*-methyl transferase (COMT) inhibitors
  — Entacapone (Comtan)

The nurse is caring for a client hospitalized with Guillain-Barré syndrome. Which information would be most important for the nurse to report to the primary healthcare provider?
A. Ascending numbness from the feet to the knees
B. A decrease in cognitive status
C. Blurred vision and sensation changes
D. A persistent unilateral headache

HESI Test Question Approach			
Positive?		YES	NO
Key Words			
Rephrase			
Rule Out Choices			
A	B	C	D

Guillain-Barré Syndrome
Involves peripheral and cranial nerves
- Usually occurs after an upper respiratory infection; surgery and vaccines are also triggers
- Acute ascending paralysis
- Rapid demyelination of the nerves
- Paralysis of the respiratory system may occur quickly.
- Prepare to intubate.
- Prolonged recovery time possible

Nursing and Collaborative Management
- Plasmapheresis over 10 to 15 days
- IV high-dose immunoglobulin (Sandoglobulin) is as effective as plasma exchange and has the advantage of immediate availability and greater safety. Clients receiving high-dose immunoglobulin need to be well hydrated and have adequate renal function.
- Maintain patent airway.
- Reposition frequently.
- Impaired swallowing may require total parenteral nutrition; nothing by mouth (NPO) if gag reflex absent.
- Supervise small frequent feedings, thicken liquids.
- Psychological support for patient and family

Multiple Sclerosis

- Demyelination of the central nervous system (CNS) myelin due to chronic inflammation
- Disease is characterized by periods of remissions and exacerbations
- Assessment findings reveal insidious onset.
  — Changes in visual field
  — Weaknesses in extremities
  — Numbness
  — Visual or swallowing difficulties
  — Severe fatigue
  — Gait disturbances

Nursing and Collaborative Management

- Encourage self-care and frequent rest periods along with physical therapy.
- Take precautions against falls.
- Voiding schedule; as incontinence worsens, teach clean self-catheterization, adequate hydration to prevent UTI.
- Bowel regimen
- Refer client for home health care and support services.
  - Administer steroid therapy and chemotherapeutic drugs in acute exacerbations to shorten attack.

Pharmacological Therapy

Focuses on controlling symptoms

- Corticosteroids (for acute exacerbations)
  — Adrenocorticotropic hormone (ACTH), prednisone, methylprednisolone
- Immunomodulators (prevent relapses)
  — Interferon-beta (Betaseron, Avonex, Rebif)
  — Glatiramer acetate (Copaxone)
- Immunosuppressants
  — Mitoxantrone hydrochloride
- Cholinergics
  — Bethanechol chloride (Duvoid [Canada]; Urecholine)
  — Neostigmine
- Anticholinergics
  — Propantheline bromide
  — Oxybutynin chloride (Ditropan)
- Muscle relaxants (for spasticity)
  — Diazepam (Valium)
  — Baclofen (Lioresal)
  — Dantrolene sodium (Dantrium)
  — Tizanidine (Zanaflex)
- CNS stimulants
  — Methylphenidate hydrochloride (Ritalin)
  — Modafinil (Alertec)
- Antiviral/antiparkinsonian drugs
  — Amantadine (Symmetrel)

Myasthenia Gravis

- A chronic neuromuscular autoimmune disease
- Caused by loss of acetylcholine (ACH) receptors in the postsynaptic neurons at the neuromuscular junction

- ACH is necessary for muscles to contract.
- Causes fluctuating weakness and abnormal fatigue of voluntary muscles; fatigue and weakness increase throughout the day

Nursing Assessment
- Ocular muscle weakness (maintaining eyes open or closed
- Bulbar muscle weakness (difficulty chewing, swallowing, or speaking)
- Skeletal muscle weakness

Diagnosis
- Based on history and clinical presentation
- Muscle weakness
- Confirmed by improved response to anticholinesterase drugs
- Tensilon test—2 mg IV

Nursing and Collaborative Management
Medications
- Anticholinesterase agents
  - Achieve maximum strength and endurance
  - Blocks action of cholinesterase
  - Increase levels of ACH at junctions
  - Common medication: pyridostigmine bromide (Mestinon)
    - Start with minimal doses.
    - Onset 30 minutes
    - Duration 3 to 4 hours
    - Must take on time!
- Corticosteroid
  - Prednisone
- Immunosuppressive agents
  - Azathioprine sodium (Imuran)
  - Cyclophosphamide (Procytox)

Types of Crises
- Myasthenic
  - Medical emergency
  - Neostigmine may be administered.
  - Caused by undermedication or infection
  - Positive Tensilon test
  - Blood pressure and pulse increase, cyanosis, loss of cough and gag reflex, incontinence
  - May require intubation
- Cholinergic
  - Results from overmedication
  - Toxic levels of anticholinesterase medications
  - Symptoms: abdominal cramps, diarrhea, excessive pulmonary secretions
  - Negative Tensilon test
  - Atropine may be administered.

Nursing and Collaborative Management
- Coughing and deep breathing exercises
- Suction equipment at bedside
- Sit upright when eating and for 1 hour afterward.
- Keep chin down when swallowing.

- Plan activities and rest carefully; weakness is greater at the end of the day.

Spinal Cord Injury
- Injuries classified by:
  - Extent of injury—complete versus incomplete
  - Level of injury—skeletal and neurologic
  - Mechanism of injury—flexion, hyperextension, flexion-rotation, extension-rotation, compression
- Rule of thumb
  - Injury above C8 = quadriplegia
  - Injury below C8 = paraplegia

Nursing Assessment
- Start with the ABCs (airway, breathing, and circulation).
- Determine quality of respiratory status.
- Check neurological status.
- Assess vital signs.
- Hypotension and bradycardia can occur in injuries above T6.

Nursing and Collaborative Management
- Immobilize and stabilize!
- Keep neck and body in anatomical alignment.
- Maintain patent airway.
- Cervical injuries are placed in skeletal traction.
- High-dose corticosteroids are used to control edema during the first 24 hours.
- Spinal shock: temporary loss of sensation, reflexes
- Flaccid paralysis/neurogenic shock
  - Complete loss of reflexes
  - Hypotension
  - Bradycardia
  - Bowel and bladder distention
- Reverse as quickly as possible.

Autonomic Dysreflexia
- Medical emergency that occurs in clients with injuries at or above T6
- Exaggerated autonomic reflex response
- Usually triggered by bowel or bladder distention
- Signs and symptoms: severe headache, ↑ BP, bradycardia, flushing, and profuse sweating
- Elevate head of bed (while maintaining correct alignment); relieve bowel or bladder distention.

Rehabilitation
- Assess for paralytic ileus.
- Kinetic bed to promote blood flow, range of motion (ROM) exercises
- Antiembolic stockings, sequential compression devices
- Assess for and protect from skin breakdown
- Bowel and bladder training
  - Keep bladder empty and urine dilute and acidic to help prevent urinary tract infection, a common cause of death after spinal cord injury.

Which action by the unlicensed assistive personnel (UAP) requires immediate follow-up by the nurse?
A. Positioning a client who is 12 hours postoperative from an above-the-knee amputation (AKA) with the residual limb elevated on a pillow
B. Assisting a client with ambulation while the client uses a cane on the unaffected side
C. Accompanying a client who has lupus erythematosus to sit outside in the sun during a break
D. Helping a client with rheumatoid arthritis to the bathroom after the client receives celecoxib (Celebrex)

HESI Test Question Approach			
Positive?		**YES**	**NO**
Key Words			
Rephrase			
Rule Out Choices			
A	**B**	**C**	**D**

Fractures

■ Signs and symptoms
  — Pain, swelling, deformity of the extremity
  — Discoloration, loss of functional ability
  — Fracture generally evident on radiograph

Nursing and Collaborative Management

■ Instruct in proper use of assistive devices.
■ Assess for the 5 Ps of neurovascular functioning:
  — Pain, paresthesia, pulse, pallor, paralysis
■ Assess neurovascular area distal to injury.
  — Skin color, temperature, sensation, capillary refill, mobility, pain, and pulses
■ Intervention
  — Closed reduction: without incision
  — Open reduction: with incision
■ Postreduction
  — Cast
  — Traction
  — External fixation
  — Splints
  — Orthoses (braces)

Joint Replacement

■ After surgery
  — Check circulation, sensation, and movement of extremity distal to replacement area.
  — Assess 5 Ps.
  — Maintain proper body alignment.
  — Encourage fluid intake.
  — Use of bed pan, commode chair
  — Coordinate rehabilitation process.
■ Discharge home
  — Safety
  — Accessibility
■ Drugs
  — Anticoagulants
  — Analgesics
  — Parenteral antibiotics

Amputation

■ Postoperative care
  — Monitor surgical dressing for drainage.

— Proper body alignment
— Elevate residual limb (stump) first 24 hours.
— Do not elevate after 48 hours.
— Provide passive ROM and encourage prone position periodically to reduce risk of contracture.
— Ensure proper stump bandaging to prepare for prosthesis.
— Coordinate care with occupational therapist, physical therapist, and social worker.
— Assess and address grieving.
■ Drug therapy
— Analgesics
  • Phantom pain is real.
— Antibiotics

The nurse is assessing a client who is scheduled for surgical fixation of a compound fracture of the right ulna. Which finding should the nurse report to the healthcare provider?
A. Ecchymosis around the fracture site
B. Crepitus at the fracture site
C. Paresthesia distal to the fracture site
D. Diminished range of motion of the right arm

HESI Test Question Approach			
Positive?		YES	NO
Key Words			
Rephrase			
Rule Out Choices			
A	B	C	D

A postmenopausal woman with a BMI of 18 has come to the clinic for her annual well-woman examination. Which teaching plan topic is most important for the nurse to prepare for this high-risk client?
A. Osteoporosis
B. Obesity
C. Anorexia
D. Breast cancer

HESI Test Question Approach			
Positive?		YES	NO
Key Words			
Rephrase			
Rule Out Choices			
A	B	C	D

Osteoporosis
Risk Factors
■ Small-boned, postmenopausal females, Caucasian, Asian, pregnancy, breastfeeding, family history
■ Diet low in calcium
■ Excessive alcohol, tobacco, and caffeine
■ Sedentary lifestyle
■ Low testosterone level (men)

Nursing Assessment
■ Dowager's hump
■ Kyphosis of the dorsal spine

- Loss of height
- Pathological fractures
- Compression fracture of the spine can occur
- Routine dual-energy X-ray absorptiometry (DEXA) screening begins at 60 years of age

Nursing and Collaborative Management

- Keep bed in low position
- Provide adequate lighting
- Avoid using throw rugs
- Provide assistance with ambulation
- Follow regular exercise program
- Diet high in vitamin D, protein, and calcium
- Vitamin D intake naturally through synthesis in the skin from exposure to sunlight; being in the sun for 20 minutes a day is generally enough

Osteoporosis Drug Therapy

- **Bisphosphonates:** require client take with only water on arising in the morning, maintaining upright in the fasting state for 30 to 60 min (120 min for tiludronate)
  — Alendronate sodium (Fosamax)
  — Etidronate disodium (Didronel)
  — Zoledronic acid (Aclasta, Zometa)
  — Ibandronate (Boniva)
  — Risedronate with calcium (Actonel Plus Calcium)
- **Selective estrogen receptor modulators** have risk for thromboembolic events
  — Raloxifene hydrochloride (Evista)
- **Recombinant parathyroid hormone:** transient hypercalcemia, joint pain are common side effects
  — Teriparatide (Forteo)

The nurse is conducting an osteoporosis screening clinic at a health fair. What information should the nurse provide to individuals who are at risk for osteoporosis? (Select all that apply.)
A. Limit alcohol and stop smoking.
B. Suggest supplementing the diet with vitamin E.
C. Promote regular weight-bearing exercise.
D. Implement a home safety plan to prevent falls.
E. Propose a regular sleep pattern of 8 hours nightly.

HESI Test Question Approach		
Positive?	YES	NO
Key Words		
Rephrase		
Rule Out Choices		
A B C D E		

Rheumatoid Arthritis

- Chronic, systemic, progressive deterioration of the connective tissue
- Etiology: unknown; believed to be autoimmune

Nursing Assessment

- Young to middle age
- More females than males
- Systemic with exacerbations and remissions

- Small joints first, then spreads
- Stiffness (may decrease with use)
- Decreased range of motion
- Joint pain
- Elevated erythrocyte sedimentation rate (ESR)
- Positive rheumatoid factor (RF) in 80% of clients
- Narrowed joint space

Nursing and Collaborative Management
Drug Therapy
- High-dose acetylsalicylic acid (ASA; aspirin) or non-steroidal antiinflammatory drugs (NSAIDs)
- Systemic corticosteroids
- Disease-modifying antirheumatic drugs (DMARDs)
  — Methotrexate (Rheumatrex)
  — Sulfasalazine (Salazopyrin [Canada]; Azulfidine)
  — Hydroxychloroquine (Plaquenil)—retinopathy risk
  — Leflunomide (Arava)

Nursing and Collaborative Management
- Heat and cold applications
- Weight management
- Rest and joint protection to maintain function
- Use assistive devices.
- Shower chair
- Canes, walkers
- Straight-back chairs, elevated seats

Lupus Erythematosus
- Two classifications
  — Discoid lupus erythematosus (DLE): affects skin only
  — Systemic lupus erythematosus (SLE): more prevalent than DLE
- Major trigger factors
  — Sunlight
  — Infectious agents
  — Stress
  — Drugs
  — Pregnancy

Nursing Assessment
- DLE: Scaly rash, butterfly rash over bridge of nose
- SLE: Joint pain, fever, nephritis, pericarditis
- Photosensitivity

Nursing and Collaborative Management
- Education
  — Drugs
  — Pain management
  — Disease process
  — Conserve energy
  — Avoid exposure to ultraviolet rays.
  — Avoid/reduce stress.
  — Use mild soaps and creams for skin care.
  — Use of steroids for joint inflammation
- Therapeutic exercise and heat therapy
- Pregnancy counseling

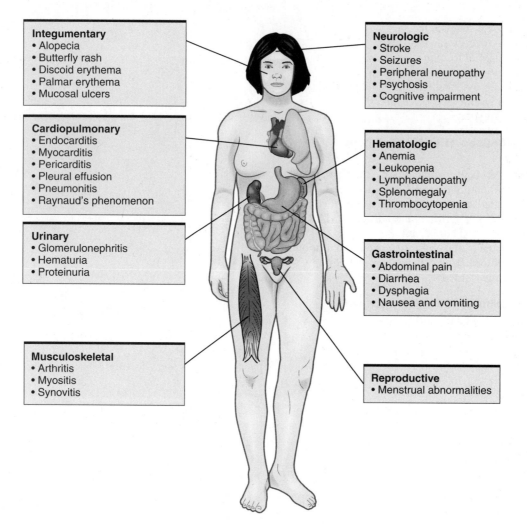

Integumentary
- Alopecia
- Butterfly rash
- Discoid erythema
- Palmar erythema
- Mucosal ulcers

Cardiopulmonary
- Endocarditis
- Myocarditis
- Pericarditis
- Pleural effusion
- Pneumonitis
- Raynaud's phenomenon

Urinary
- Glomerulonephritis
- Hematuria
- Proteinuria

Musculoskeletal
- Arthritis
- Myositis
- Synovitis

Neurologic
- Stroke
- Seizures
- Peripheral neuropathy
- Psychosis
- Cognitive impairment

Hematologic
- Anemia
- Leukopenia
- Lymphadenopathy
- Splenomegaly
- Thrombocytopenia

Gastrointestinal
- Abdominal pain
- Diarrhea
- Dysphagia
- Nausea and vomiting

Reproductive
- Menstrual abnormalities

Figure 8-1 Common assessment findings in SLE (From Lewis, S., Dirksen, S., Heitkemper M, et al. *Medical-surgical nursing: Assessment and management of clinical problems*, 8th ed St. Louis, 2011, Mosby.)

Kidney involvement is the leading cause of death in clients with lupus; the second leading cause is cardiac involvement.

Degenerative Joint Disease (Osteoarthritis)

- Joint pain—increases with activity
- Morning stiffness
- Crepitus
- Limited movement
- Joint enlargement

Nursing and Collaborative Management

- Weight reduction diet
- Excessive use of involved joint may accelerate degeneration
- Use proper body mechanics.
- Keep joints in functional position.
- Hot and cold applications for pain and stiffness
- NSAIDs, opioid analgesics, and intraarticular corticosteroids

The nurse observes an elderly male client with glaucoma administer eyedrops by tilting his head back, instilling each drop close to the inner canthus, and keeping his eye closed for 15 seconds. What action should the nurse take first?

A. Ask the client whether another family member is available to administer the drops.
B. Review the correct steps of the procedure with the client.
C. Administer the eyedrops correctly in the other eye to demonstrate the technique.
D. Discuss the importance of correct eyedrop administration for persons with glaucoma.

HESI Test Question Approach			
Positive?		YES	NO
Key Words			
Rephrase			
Rule Out Choices			
A	B	C	D

Glaucoma

- Primary open-angle glaucoma—more common
  — Drainage channels become clogged.
  — Aqueous humor flow is reduced in trabecular meshwork.
- Primary closure-angle glaucoma—painful if acute
  — Bulging lens from age-related processes disrupts flow.
- Silent thief of vision
- Normally painless until later stages
- Loss of peripheral vision
- May see halos around lights
- Diagnosed with eye examination
  — Tonometer to measure intraocular pressure

Nursing and Collaborative Management

- Keys to treatment
  — ↓ Intraocular pressure; normal limits is 10 to 21 mm Hg
  — ↓ Aqueous humor production
  — ↑ Drainage of aqueous humor
  — Teach client proper eyedrop instillation
  — Teach client to avoid activities that can increase intraocular pressure
- Ambulatory/home care for open-angle glaucoma
  — Drug therapy
    • Beta-adrenergic blockers
    • Alpha-adrenergic agonists
    • Cholinergic agents (miotics): decrease visual acuity in low-light environments
    • Carbonic anhydrase inhibitors
  — Surgical therapy
  — Argon laser trabeculoplasty (ALT)
  — Trabeculectomy with or without filtering implant
- Acute care for closure-angle glaucoma
  — Topical cholinergic agent
  — Hyperosmotic agent
  — Laser peripheral iridotomy
  — Surgical iridectomy

Glaucoma Drug Therapy

- Beta-adrenergic blockers

- — Betaxolol hydrochloride (Betoptic)
- — Timolol maleate (Apo-Timop [Canada]; Timoptic, Istalol)
- Alpha-adrenergic agonists
  - — Dipivefrin hydrochloride (Propine)
  - — Epinephryl (Epinal)
- Cholinergic agents (miotics)
  - — Carbachol (Miostat)
  - — Pilocarpine hydrochloride (Akarpine, Diocarpine, Minims [Canada], Isopto Carpine, Pilocar)
- Carbonic anhydrase inhibitors
  - — Systemic
    - Acetazolamide (Acetazolam [Canada]; Diamox)
    - Methazolamide
  - — Topical
    - Brinzolamide (Azopt)
    - Dorzolamide (Trusopt)
- Combination therapy
  - — Timolol maleate and dorzolamide (Cosopt)
- Hyperosmolar agents
  - — Glycerin liquid
  - — Mannitol solution (Osmitrol)

Cataracts
- Clouding or opacity of the lens
- Early signs
  - — Blurred vision
  - — Decreased color perception
- Late signs
  - — Double vision
  - — Clouded pupil

Nursing and Collaborative Management: Cataract Removal
- Preoperative
  - — Assess medications being taken.
  - — Anticoagulants should be stopped before surgery.
  - — Teach how to instill eyedrops.
- Postoperative
  - — Eye shield should be worn during sleeping hours.
  - — Avoid lifting >10 lb.
  - — Avoid lying on operative side.
  - — Report signs of increased intraocular pressure.
  - — Acute pain abnormal finding

The nurse is teaching an 86-year-old client who has glaucoma and bilateral hearing loss. Which intervention should the nurse implement?

A. Maintain constant eye contact.
B. Stand on the side unaffected by glaucoma.
C. Speak in a lower tone of voice.
D. Keep the environment dimly lit.

HESI Test Question Approach			
Positive?		YES	NO
Key Words			
Rephrase			
Rule Out Choices			
A	B	C	D

Eye Trauma/Injury
- Trauma
  - Determine type of injury.
  - Position client in sitting position to decrease intra-ocular pressure.
  - Never attempt to remove embedded object.
  - Irrigate eye if a chemical injury has occurred.
- Detached retina
  - Described as curtain falling over visual field
  - Painless
  - May have black spots or floaters (indicates bleeding has occurred with detachment)
  - Surgical repair of retina
  - Keep eye patch over affected area.

Hearing Loss
- Conductive hearing loss
  - Sounds do not travel to the inner ear
  - May benefit from hearing aid
- Sensorineural hearing loss
  - Sound distorted from defect in inner ear
- Common causes
  - Infections
  - Ototoxic drugs
    - Gentamicin
    - Vancomycin
    - Lasix
  - Trauma
  - Aging process
- Assessment
  - Inability to hear whisper from 1 to 2 feet
  - Shouting in conversations
  - Turning head to favor one ear
  - Loud volume on TV or radio

A client with a history of myasthenia gravis presents with a heart rate of 112 beats/min, respiration rate 24/min with accessory muscle use, anxiety, and restlessness. Which of these interventions demonstrate best practice? (Select all that apply).

A. Elevate the head of the bed to 45-degree angle.
B. Prepare to administer Lasix 40 mg IV.
C. Administer 2 L of oxygen per prescription.
D. Teach the importance of wearing a medical ID bracelet.
E. Apply lubricating eyedrops to both eyes.

HESI Test Question Approach			
Positive?		YES	NO
Key Words			
Rephrase			
Rule Out Choices			
A	B	C	D	E

9 Pediatric Nursing

The nurse directs the unlicensed assistive personnel (UAP) to play with a 4-year-old child on bed rest. Which activity should the nurse recommend? Select all that apply.

A. Monopoly board game
B. Looking at picture books
C. Fifty-piece puzzle
D. Hand puppets
E. Coloring book

HESI Test Question Approach		
Positive?	**YES**	**NO**
Key Words		
Rephrase		
Rule Out Choices		
A	**B**	**C** **D** **E**

Growth and Development

- Five major developmental periods
  — Infant
  — Toddler
  — Preschool
  — School Age
  — Adolescent
- Developmental theories most widely used to explain child's growth and development
  — Freud's psychosexual stages
  — Erikson's stages of psychosocial development
  — Piaget's stages of cognitive development
  — Kohlberg's stages of moral development

Normal Growth and Development

Know norms for growth and development
- Infant (birth to 1 year)
  — Birth weight doubles by 6 months, triples by 12 months.
  — Social smile occurs at 2 months.
  — Plays "peek-a-boo" by 6 months
  — Sits upright without support by 8 months
  — Develops separation anxiety at 6 months
  — Fine pincer grasp by 10 to 12 months (can pick up Cheerios)
  — Crawls by 9 months
  — Walking with support—11 months to 1 year
  — Says a few words in addition to "mama" or "dada" at 12 months
- Toddler (1 to 3 years)
  — Two- to three-word sentences at 2 years
  — Toilet training starts around 2 years
  — Ritualistic
  — No concept of time
  — Frequent tantrums

- Preschool-age child (3 to 5 years)
  - Favorite word: *Why?*
  - Sentences of five to eight words
- School-age child (6 to 12 years)
  - Each year gains 4 to 6 lb, grows 2 inches.
  - Socialization with peers very important
- Adolescent (12 to 19 years)
  - Rapid growth, second only to the first year of life
  - Secondary sex characteristics develop

A parent is preparing her or his 5-year-old child for kindergarten. The child has not had any immunizations. What vaccines will be given to start school? Select all that apply.
A. DTaP
B. Inactivated polio virus (IPV)
C. Varicella
D. Pneumococcal conjugate vaccine (PCV)
E. Trivalent inactivated influenza vaccine (TIV)

HESI Test Question Approach		
Positive?	YES	NO
Key Words		
Rephrase		
Rule Out Choices		
A B C D E		

A 7-year-old is to have a painful procedure. Which statement by the nurse best prepares the child to cope with this?
A. "It feels like burning pain."
B. "Sometimes this feels like pushing."
C. "There is nothing wrong when you have pain."
D. "You will get ice cream after the procedure."

HESI Test Question Approach		
Positive?	YES	NO
Key Words		
Rephrase		
Rule Out Choices		
A B C D		

Pain Assessment and Management
- Assessment is based on verbal and nonverbal cues from child's and parents' information.
- Be aware of developmental responses to pain (i.e., intense, sustained crying in infants).
- Use appropriate pain scale.
- Safety is the priority in administering medication.
- Make sure dose is safe for age and weight.

Nursing Interventions
Nonpharmacological Interventions
- Infants may respond best to pacifiers, holding, rocking and oral sucrose.
- Toddlers and preschoolers may respond best to distraction.
- School-age children and adolescents may use guided imagery.

Pharmacological Interventions

- Before administering a pain medication to a pediatric client, verify that the prescribed dose is safe for the child on the basis of the child's weight.
- Monitor the child's vital signs before and after administration of opioid medications.
- Children as young as 5 years of age may be taught to use a patient-controlled analgesia (PCA) pump.

Immunization Teaching

- To prepare for NCLEX-RN exam, use knowledge from the immunization chart: *http://www.cdc.gov/vaccines/schedules/index.html*.
- *Example:* What vaccines would the nurse expect to be prescribed for a 2-month-old brought into the pediatrician's office for a well-baby checkup?

  Answer: DTaP, HepB, HIB, IPV, and PCV
- *Example:* Withhold MMR vaccine for a person with a history of an anaphylactic reaction to neomycin or eggs.
- Common cold does *not* contraindicate immunization unless the fever is >37.2 °C (99 °F)
- A fever <38.9 °C (<102 °F) and redness and soreness at the injection site are normal for 2 to 3 days after vaccination.
- Call healthcare provider if child has high-pitched crying, seizures, or high fever.
- Use acetaminophen orally, before and every 4 to 6 hours after immunization for 24 hours.

Communicable Diseases

The incidence of common childhood communicable diseases has declined greatly since the advent of immunizations, but they do occur, and nurses should be able to identify the infection.

- Measles
- Rubeola
- Rubella
- Roseola
- Mumps
- Pertussis
- Diphtheria
- Varicella
- Erythema infectiosum (fifth disease)
- Treat fever from infection with acetaminophen, *not* ASA (acetylsalicylic acid, aspirin)
- Isolation is required during the infectious phase of the disease.
- Teaching is the primary intervention for the prevention of spread.
- Handwashing
- Provide supportive measures while the disease runs its course.

Poisonings

- Frequent cause of childhood injury—teach poison-proofing methods for the home
- Children less than 6 with a peak at 2 years of age

- Gastrointestinal (GI) disturbance is a common symptom.
- Burns of the mouth and pharynx with caustic poisonings
- Identify poisonous agent quickly.
- Check ABCs (airway, breathing, and circulation).
- Teach parents not to make child vomit because this may cause more damage.
- Call Poison Control Center or 911, depending on how the child is acting.

The nurse is performing the initial assessment of a 2-year-old child with suspected bacterial epiglottitis. Which technique is needed?
A. Use a tongue depressor to assess for erythema.
B. Obtain a throat swab for culture and sensitivity.
C. Observe for the presence of drooling.
D. Measure pain using a FACES scale.

Respiratory Dysfunction

- Infections of the respiratory tract
- Croup syndromes
- Tuberculosis
- Asthma
- Cystic fibrosis

A nurse is caring for a 6-year-old child who had a tonsillectomy 2 hours ago. Which sign or symptom most likely relates to a complication?
A. Apical rate 90 beats/min
B. Blood pressure 96/50
C. Frequent swallowing
D. Nasal congestion

HESI Test Question Approach			
Positive?		**YES**	**NO**
Key Words			
Rephrase			
Rule Out Choices			
A	B	C	D

HESI Test Question Approach			
Positive?		**YES**	**NO**
Key Words			
Rephrase			
Rule Out Choices			
A	B	C	D

A 4-year-old is brought to the clinic with a fever of 39.4 °C (103 °F), sore throat, and moderate respiratory distress caused by a suspected bacterial infection. Which medical diagnosis is a contraindication to obtaining a throat culture in the child?

A. Tonsillitis
B. Streptococcal infection
C. Bronchiolitis
D. Epiglottitis

HESI Test Question Approach			
Positive?		**YES**	**NO**
Key Words			
Rephrase			
Rule Out Choices			
A	B	C	D

The nurse is completing discharge teaching on a 2-year-old child with active tuberculosis. Which instruction(s) should the nurse provide to the family member? Select all that apply.

A. Inform the family that bodily fluids may turn an orange-red color.
B. Stress the importance of adequate nap and sleep time.
C. Advise the family to wear gloves when cleansing the child's face and nose.
D. Place the child in home isolation until medications are completed.
E. Avoid contact with other individuals, except family members, for at least 6 months.

HESI Test Question Approach				
Positive?			**YES**	**NO**
Key Words				
Rephrase				
Rule Out Choices				
A	B	C	D	E

Respiratory Disorders

- Be familiar with normal values for respiratory and pulse rates for children.
- Cardinal signs of respiratory distress
  — Restlessness
  — Increased respiratory rate
  — Increased pulse rate, tachypnea, nasal flaring, grunting, intercostal retractions, and cyanosis occur in newborn.
- Respiratory failure usually occurs before cardiac failure.

Respiratory Infections

- Nasopharyngitis
- Tonsillitis
- May be viral or bacterial
- Treatment is important if related to streptococcal infection
- Surgical treatment
  — Check prothrombin time (PT) and partial thromboplastin time (PTT) before surgery.
  — Monitor for bleeding.
  — Highest risk for bleeding is during first 24 hours and 5 to 10 days postoperative.
- Otitis media
- Signs/symptoms: fever, pulling at ear
- Discharge from ear

- Administer antibiotics if prescribed; now not always prescribed.
- Position on affected side.
- Reduce temperature to prevent seizures.
- Bronchitis—inflammation of the trachea and bronchi
  — Rhinitis and cough
  — Crackles and rhonchi
  — Symptomatic treatment
- Respiratory syncytial virus bronchiolitis
- Isolate child (contact isolation).
- Monitor respiratory status and maintain patent airway.
- Antiviral agent (ribavirin aerosols)
- Respiratory syncytial virus prophylaxis with monoclonal antibody palivizumab (Synagis) in high-risk children <2 years old
- Epiglottitis
- Signs/symptoms: high fever, sore throat, muffled voice, tripod position
- Intravenous (IV) antibiotics
- Do not examine throat; this may cause complete airway obstruction.
- Be prepared for tracheostomy.

Croup
- Primarily viral infection
- Hoarseness, brassy or barky cough, varying degrees of respiratory distress; worse at night
- Supportive measures—in cool mist humidity
- Increased oral intake
- Oral dexamethasone

Tuberculosis. See Chapter 5.
Asthma
- Leading cause of chronic illness in children
- Allergies influence persistence and severity.
- Complex disorder involving biochemical, immunological, infection, endocrine, and psychological factors

Nursing Assessment and Interventions
- Signs/symptoms: Tight cough, expiratory wheezing, decreased peak flow levels
- Monitor for respiratory distress, need for O_2 nebulizer therapy.
- Rescue versus maintenance medications
- Evaluate effects of beta-adrenergic agonists, such as albuterol, and salbutamol sulfate and levalbuterol [Xopenex], as well as antiinflammatory corticosteroids.

The nurse is teaching the school-age child and parent about the administration of inhaled beclomethasone dipropionate and ipratropium bromide for the treatment of asthma. Which statement by the parent indicates that teaching has been effective?

A. "I'll keep the inhalers in the refrigerator."
B. "My child only needs to use the inhalers when the peak flow numbers are in the red."
C. "My child will take the bronchodilator first, then the corticosteroid."
D. "My child will take the corticosteroid first, wait a few minutes, and then take the bronchodilator."

HESI Test Question Approach			
Positive?		**YES**	**NO**
Key Words			
Rephrase			
Rule Out Choices			
A	**B**	**C**	**D**

Cystic Fibrosis (CF)

- Most frequently occurring as an inherited disease of Caucasian children
- Transmitted by an autosomal recessive gene
- Chronic multisystem disorder
- Abnormally thick mucus; primarily lung and pancreatic involvement
- Positive newborn screening test
- First sign may be meconium ileus at birth.
- High sweat chloride concentration (pilocarpine test or sweat test)
- Delayed growth, poor weight gain
- Pancreatic enzymes with each meal and snacks, fat-soluble vitamins
- Teach family percussion and postural drainage techniques.

Cardiovascular Disorders

Congenital Heart Disorders

May be classified as acyanotic or cyanotic. Most important is the management of the symptoms.

For descriptions and illustrations of congenital cardiovascular disorders, see a textbook or an NCLEX review manual:

- *Evolve Reach Comprehensive Review for the NCLEX-RN Examination* (powered by HESI)
- *Mosby's Comprehensive Review of Nursing for the NCLEX-RN Examination*
- *Saunders Comprehensive Review for the NCLEX-RN Examination Nursing and Collaborative Management*

Congestive Heart Failure

- Common complication of congenital heart disorders
- Signs/symptoms: pedal edema, neck vein distention, respiratory distress, fatigue, irritability, sudden weight gain
- Monitor vital signs, elevate head of bed, O_2
- Digoxin, diuretics, and angiotensin-converting enzyme (ACE) inhibitors
- Weigh daily on same scale
- Maintain nutritional status; feeding should not last >30 minutes.
- Plan frequent rest periods.

Managing Digoxin Therapy in Children

- Count apical rate when child is at rest; withhold medication if pulse is <90 to 110 beats/min in infants or <70 beats/min in older children.
- Notify healthcare provider.
- Do not skip or try to make up doses.
- Give 1 to 2 hours before meals.
- Watch for signs/symptoms of toxicity and teach them to parents: vomiting, diarrhea, anorexia, muscle weakness and drowsiness.
- Provide adequate potassium in the diet.

Rheumatic Fever

- Peaks in school-age children
- Most common cause of acquired heart disease.
- Affects connective tissue
- Signs/symptoms: Sore throat appears to be getting better (typically follows a group A *Streptococcus* infection), and then fever develops along with rash, chorea, and elevated erythrocyte sedimentation rate.
- Antibiotic prophylaxis for invasive procedures

Nursing and Collaborative Management

- Encourage compliance with drug regimens.
- Penicillin remains drug of choice.
- Salicylates are used to control inflammatory process and to reduce fever and discomfort.
- Prednisone may be indicated in some clients with heart failure.
- Bed rest or at least limited activity during acute illness
- Provide emotional support.

A 13-month-old with a congenital heart defect is prescribed digoxin. The maintenance dosage ordered by the healthcare provider (HCP) is 50 mcg/kg/day, and the child weighs 10 kg. The HCP prescribes the digoxin to be given twice daily. The nurse prepares how much digoxin to administer to the client at each dose? (Fill in the blank.)

_____

A 2-year-old child is prescribed furosemide, digoxin, and captopril for congestive heart failure. Which value should the nurse verify with the laboratory?
A. Increased serum calcium level
B. Reduced serum sodium level
C. Low hemoglobin level
D. Low serum potassium level

HESI Test Question Approach			
Positive?		YES	NO
Key Words			
Rephrase			
Rule Out Choices			
A	B	C	D

The nurse is caring for a 3-month-old child with congestive heart failure. Which sign or symptom most clearly relates to a side effect of furosemide?
A. Increased skin turgor
B. Decreased urine output
C. Bulging fontanels
D. Peripheral edema

HESI Test Question Approach			
Positive?		**YES**	**NO**
Key Words			
Rephrase			
Rule Out Choices			
A	B	C	D

The nurse reviews the medication record of a 2-month-old and notes that the infant was given a scheduled dose of digoxin with a documented apical pulse of 76 beats/min. What action should the nurse take first?
A. Assess the current apical heart rate.
B. Observe for the onset of diarrhea.
C. Complete an adverse occurrence report.
D. Determine the serum potassium level.

HESI Test Question Approach			
Positive?		**YES**	**NO**
Key Words			
Rephrase			
Rule Out Choices			
A	B	C	D

A child with hydrocephalus is 1 day postoperative for revision of a ventriculoatrial shunt. Which finding is most important?
A. Increased blood pressure
B. Increased temperature
C. Increased serum glucose
D. Increased hematocrit

HESI Test Question Approach			
Positive?		**YES**	**NO**
Key Words			
Rephrase			
Rule Out Choices			
A	B	C	D

Neuromuscular Disorders

The nurse is caring for a 16-year-old client with Down syndrome who has a mental age of 5 in the acute care hospital. Which priority nursing action should be included in this client's plan of care?

A. Monitoring for hearing loss
B. Monitoring intake and output (I & O)
C. Providing a dependable routine
D. Providing small puzzles

HESI Test Question Approach		
Positive?	**YES**	**NO**
Key Words		
Rephrase		
Rule Out Choices		
A	**B**	**C**	**D**

Down Syndrome

- Flat, broad nasal bridge; upward, outward slanting eyes
- Commonly associated problems
- Cardiac defects
- Delayed development
- Respiratory infections
- Feed to back and side of mouth due to tongue thrust
- Support child/parent relationship to achieve the highest level of functioning
- Always evaluate mental age
- Refer family to early intervention program

Cerebral Palsy (CP)

- Diagnosis made on evaluation of child
- Permanent injury to the motor centers of the brain before, during, or after birth
- Persistent neonatal reflexes after 6 months—no parachute reflex
- Spasticity
- Muscle and motor tone abnormalities

Nursing and Collaborative Management

- Prevent aspiration with feedings.
- Phenytoin for seizures
- Diazepam for muscle spasms
- Botulinum toxin A for muscle stiffness

Spina Bifida Occulta

- No sac present
- Suspect if tuft of hair at base of spine

Meningocele

- Sac contains only meninges and spinal fluid.
- No nerves in spinal sac

Myelomeningocele

- Sac contains spinal fluid, meninges, and nerves.
- Client has sensory and motor defects.
- Preoperative/postoperative care
- Monitor urine output.
- Watch for ↑ intracranial pressure (ICP).
- Keep sac free of stool and urine.
- Measure head circumference every 8 hours and check fontanels.

Hydrocephalus

- Abnormal accumulation of cerebrospinal fluid (CSF)
- Symptoms
- ↑ ICP
- ↑ Blood pressure
- ↓ Pulse
- Changes in level of consciousness
- Irritability and vomiting
- Shrill high-pitched cry in infants

Nursing and Collaborative Management

- Elevate head of bed.
- Seizure precautions
- Prepare for shunt placement.
- Assess for shunt malfunctioning.
- Monitor for signs/symptoms of infection.
- Teaching related to shunt replacement

Seizures/Epilepsy

- Uncontrolled electrical activity of neurons
- More common in children under 2 years
- Types of seizures
  - Generalized
    - Tonic/clonic (formerly grand mal)
    - Aura
    - Loss of consciousness
    - Tonic phase: stiffness of body
    - Clonic phase: spasms and relaxation
    - Postictal phase: sleepy and disoriented
  - Absence seizures (formerly petit mal)
    - Momentary loss of consciousness, appears like daydreaming, poor performance in school
    - Lasts 5 to 30 seconds
  - Partial seizures
    - Specific area in the brain; limited symptoms
  - Status epilepticus
    - Series of seizures at intervals too brief to allow the child to regain consciousness

Nursing and Collaborative Management: Seizures

- Maintain patent airway.
- Side rails up
- Pad side rails.
- Do not use tongue blade.
- Administer anticonvulsants.
- Teach family/client about medication.

Anticonvulsants/Types of Seizures

- Phenobarbital
  - Generalized tonic clonic
  - Partial
  - Status epilepticus
- Primidone
  - Generalized tonic clonic
  - Partial
  - Status epilepticus
- Phenytoin
  - Generalized tonic clonic
  - Partial
  - Status epilepticus

- Fosphenytoin sodium intramuscular (IM), IV
  — Generalized convulsive status epilepticus
  — Treatment of seizures during neurosurgery
  — Short-term parenteral replacement for phenytoin oral
- Valproic acid
  — Generalized tonic clonic
  — Absence
  — Myoclonic
  — Partial
- Clonazepam
  — Absence
  — Myoclonic
  — Infantile spasms
  — Partial
- Carbamazepine
  — Generalized tonic-clonic
  — Partial

Bacterial Meningitis
- Usually caused by *Haemophilus influenzae* type B, *Streptococcus pneumoniae*, and *Neisseria meningitidis*. Enteric bacilli and group B *Streptococcus* for infants
- Signs and symptoms
  — Petechial or purpuric rashes (meningococcal infection), especially when associated with shock-like state
  — Older children: include signs and symptoms of increased ICP, neck stiffness, positive Kernig's sign, positive Brudzinski's sign
  — Infants: classic signs absent; poor feeding, vomiting, irritability, bulging fontanels
- Diagnostic procedures include lumbar puncture for laboratory analysis.

Nursing and Collaborative Management
- Isolate at least 24 hours.
- Administer antibiotics.
- Frequent vital signs and neurological checks
- Increased ICP, muscle twitching, and changes in level of consciousness
- Measure head circumference daily.
- Syndrome of inappropriate antidiuretic hormone (SIADH) occurs frequently.
- Fluid restrictions may be necessary.

Reye's Syndrome
- Etiology often, but not always, associated with aspirin use and influenza or varicella
- Rapidly progressing encephalopathy
- Altered hepatic function
- Signs/symptoms: lethargy progressing to coma, vomiting, hypoglycemia
- Neurological checks; maintain airway
- Mannitol for ICP control
- Early diagnosis is important to improve client outcome.

Muscular Dystrophy (MD)
- Duchenne's MD
- Onset between ages 2 and 6 years
- Most severe and most common MD of childhood

- X-linked recessive disorder
- Diagnosis
- Muscle biopsy muscle fibers degenerate and are replaced by connective tissue and fat.
- Serum creatine phosphokinase (CK) levels are extremely high in the first 2 years of life before the onset.
- Symptoms
- Delayed walking
- Frequent falls
- Easily tires when walking
- Interventions
- Exercise
- Prevent falls
- Assistive devices for ambulation
- Loss of ambulation 8 to 12 years old

Renal Disorders in Children

Urinary Tract Infection (UTI)
- More common in girls
- Symptoms
- Poor food intake
- Strong-smelling urine
- Fever
- Pain with urination
- Interventions
- Obtain urine culture before starting antibiotics.
- Teach home care.
- Finish all antibiotics.
- Avoid bubble baths.
- Increase intake of fluids.

Acute Glomerulonephritis (AGN)
- Common features
- Oliguria, hematuria, and proteinuria
- Edema
- Hypertension
- Circulatory congestion
- Therapeutic management
- Maintenance of fluid balance
- Treatment of hypertension
- Assessment
- Recent strep infection
- Dark ("iced tea") urine
- Irritable and/or lethargic

Nursing and Collaborative Management
- Vital signs every 4 hours or as prescribed
- Daily weights
- Low-sodium, low-potassium diet
- Usually recover without long-term effects

Nephrotic Syndrome
- Characterized by increased glomerular permeability to protein
- Assessment
- Frothy urine
- Massive proteinuria
- Edema
- Anorexia

Nursing and Collaborative Management

- Reducing excretion of protein
- Reducing or preventing fluid retention
- Preventing infection
- Skin care
- Administer medications.
- Diuretics: characteristic of disease a usual lack of responsiveness to diuretics
- If infections develop, antibiotics
- Corticosteroid therapy
- Immunosuppressants
- Small frequent feeding

Discharge Teaching

- Daily weights
- Side effects of meds, i.e., growth retardation from steroids
- Prevent infections.

Renal Failure Management. See Chapter 7.

A school-age child with nephrotic syndrome has just received hemodialysis. Which assessment is most important to obtain after hemodialysis?
A. Pain assessment
B. Capillary refill
C. Urine ketones
D. Daily weight

HESI Test Question Approach			
Positive?		**YES**	**NO**
Key Words			
Rephrase			
Rule Out Choices			
A	**B**	**C**	**D**

Gastrointestinal Disorders

Nutritional Assessment

- Present nutritional status
- Body mass index
- Dietary history
- Past nutrition assessment
- Height
- Weight
- Head circumference
- Skinfold thickness
- Arm circumference
- Iron deficiency
- $FeSO_4$ drops: use straw; give with orange juice, not with dairy foods

Diarrhea

- Worldwide leading cause of death in children <5 years of age
- Classified as acute or chronic
- Common problem for infants
- Assessment
- Depressed sunken eyes
- Weight loss
- Decreased urine output

Nursing and Collaborative Management

- Fluid and electrolyte balance
- Rehydration
- Maintenance fluid therapy
- Reintroduction of adequate diet
- Do not give antidiarrheal agents.

Cleft Lip or Cleft Palate

- Malformation of the face or oral cavity
- Initial closure of cleft lip is performed when infant is approximately 3 months of age.
- Closure of cleft palate at around 9 to 15 months
- Promote bonding
- Breck/Haberman feeder and slow-flow nipple
- Maintain airway.
- No straws, no spoons, only soft foods for cleft palate

Pyloric Stenosis

- Common in firstborn males
- Vomiting becomes projectile around day 14 after birth
- Dehydration, weight loss, and failure to thrive

Perioperative Care of Client for Repair Intussusception

- Telescoping of one part of intestine
- Emergency intervention is needed; necrosis and perforation of the bowel
- Sudden onset of crampy abdominal pain, inconsolable crying, and drawing knees up to chest in an otherwise healthy child

Congenital Aganglionic Megacolon (Hirschsprung's Disease)

- Series of surgeries to correct
- Temporary colostomy and then at 6 to 12 months a rectal pull through

Hematological Disorders

Sickle Cell Anemia

- Autosomal recessive disorder
- Fetal hemoglobin does not sickle.
- Hydration to promote hemodilution
- Symptoms
  — Crisis marked by fever and pain
- Treatment during crisis
  — Bedrest to minimize energy expenditure
  — Improve oxygen utilization.
  — Hydration through oral and IV therapy
  — Analgesia for severe pain from vaso-occlusion
  — Blood replacement to treat anemia and to reduce the viscosity of the sickled blood
  — Antibiotic therapy to treat any existing infection
- Maintenance
  — Keep well hydrated.
  — Do not give supplemental iron.
  — Give folic acid orally.
  — Start penicillin prophylactically at 2 months of age to decrease risk of pneumococcal pneumonia infection.

Hemophilia

- X-linked recessive disorder; deficiency of specific clotting factors
- Interventions
  — Replacement of missing clotting factor (i.e., factor VIII concentrates)
  — Apply pressure to even minor bleeding.
- Increased risk for bleeding

Metabolic and Endocrine Disorders

Phenylketonuria (PKU)

- Autosomal recessive disorder
- Newborn screening for inborn errors of metabolism
- Performed at birth after 24 hours of age
- Strict adherence to low-phenylalanine diet; prevents mental retardation
- Avoid meat, dairy, and aspartame-containing foods and drinks.
- Use: fruits, juices, cereal, bread, and starches

Diabetes

Obesity

- 19% of 6- to 11-year-olds categorized as overweight or obese
- Leads to adult obesity with increased risks of cardiovascular issues and type 2 diabetes
- Minorities disproportionally at risk
- Parental obesity is the highest predictor of childhood obesity.
- Body mass index (BMI), dietary, and activity assessments should be obtained and evaluated.

Type 2 diabetes: The defect is insulin resistance and relative insulin deficiency. There is insufficient insulin production, insulin resistance, and/or excessive and unregulated glucose production from the liver.
- Risk of overweight: BMI-for-age 85th percentile
- Overweight: BMI-for-age >95th percentile
- Acanthosis nigricans (a marker) is a risk factor for diabetes.

Type 1 diabetes: Immune-mediated disease associated with absolute insulin deficiency. The body's own T cells destroy pancreatic beta cells, which are the source of insulin. Type 1 diabetes is common in school-age children. Classic symptoms are polyuria, polyphagia, polydipsia, and weight loss. Child may wet the bed. Cognitive level and age should be considered when planning teaching.
- Dietary teaching
- Exercise management
- Insulin administration
- Continuous follow-up important
- Monitoring
- Hypoglycemia

Skeletal Disorders

Nursing Assessment

- Visible signs of fractures
- Obtain baseline pulses, color, movement, sensation, temperature, swelling, and pain or 5 Ps—pallor, paresthesias, pain, paralysis, and pulses.
- Report any changes immediately.

Traction

Fractures not easily reduced by casting and for presurgical stabilization of fracture

- Buck's traction
- For knee immobilization
- Russell's traction
- For fracture of femur or lower leg
- Can be skeletal or skin
- 90 degree/90 degree traction
- Pinned for desired line of pull and flexion at hip and knee of 90 degrees
- Provide appropriate toys, teach cast care to family, prevent cast soilage with diapering, and monitor neurovascular status.

Congenital Dislocated Hip

- Assessment
- Positive Ortolani's sign
- Unequal fold of skin on buttocks
- Limited abduction of hip

Nursing and Collaborative Management

- Apply Pavlik harness (worn 24 hours a day) for up to 6 months.
- Surgical correction after 6 months closed reduction and hip spica cast if nonoperative treatment is not effective
- Postoperative intervention
- Hip spica cast care

Scoliosis

- S-shaped curvature of the spine
- Most common nontraumatic skeletal condition in children
- Milwaukee brace
- Affects both genders at all ages but is most commonly seen in adolescents

Juvenile Idiopathic Arthritis (JIA)

- Most common chronic arthritic condition of childhood
- Inflammatory diseases that involve the joints, connective tissues, and viscera
- Exact cause unknown, but infections and autoimmune response have been implicated
- Therapy consists of administration of medications (e.g., NSAIDs, methotrexate, biological agents, and interleukin-1), along with exercise, heat application, and support of joints.

The practical nurse (PN) is assigned by the RN charge nurse to care for a 3-year-old with Reye's syndrome. The child's temperature is 39.1 °C (102.4 °F), and the PN is preparing to administer aspirin PO. What action should the charge nurse implement?

A. Direct the PN to assess the gag reflex and level of consciousness.
B. Advise the PN to wait until the fever is greater than 39.1 °C (102.4 °F).
C. Remind the PN to hold all aspirin-containing medications.
D. Tell the PN to notify the healthcare provider.

HESI Test Question Approach			
Positive?		YES	NO
Key Words			
Rephrase			
Rule Out Choices			
A	B	C	D

While receiving IV antibiotics for sepsis, a 2-month-old is crying inconsolably despite the mother's presence. The nurse recognizes that the infant is exhibiting symptoms related to which condition?

A. Allergic reaction to the antibiotics
B. Pain related to IV infiltration
C. Separation anxiety from the mother
D. Hunger and thirst

HESI Test Question Approach			
Positive?		YES	NO
Key Words			
Rephrase			
Rule Out Choices			
A	B	C	D

A client at 36 weeks' gestation is placed in the lithotomy position; she suddenly complains of feeling breathless and lightheaded and shows marked pallor. What action should the nurse take first?

A. Turn her to a lateral position.
B. Place her in the Trendelenburg position.
C. Obtain vital signs and a pulse oximetry reading.
D. Initiate distraction techniques.

HESI Test Question Approach			
Positive?		YES	NO
Key Words			
Rephrase			
Rule Out Choices			
A	B	C	D

Pregnancy: Key Assessments

- Assess for violence
  - Battering and emotional or physical abuse can begin with pregnancy, higher risk of homicide
  - Assess for abuse in private, away from the partner, throughout pregnancy.
  - Nurse needs to know:
    - Local resources
    - How to determine client's safety
- Gravidity and parity count pregnancies, not offspring
  - *Gravida:* Number of times woman has been pregnant, including current pregnancy, regardless of outcome
  - *Para:* Number of deliveries (not children) occurring after 20 weeks of gestation
    - Multiple births count as one gravida or para.
    - Pregnancy loss before 20 weeks counted as abortion but add 1 to gravidity
    - Fetal demise after 20 weeks is added to parity.
- GTPAL represents obstetric history
  G Gravidity: number of pregnancies
  T Term pregnancies: after 37 weeks
  P Preterm pregnancies: before 37 weeks.
  A Abortions (elective or spontaneous): loss before 20 weeks.
  L Living children
- Gestation
  - Naegele's rule
    - Count back 3 months from date of last normal menstrual period
    - Add 1 year and 7 days

Example: If the last menstrual period was May 2, 2015, estimated date of birth would be February 9, 2016.

- Fundal height
  - 12 to 13 weeks: Fundus rises out of symphysis.
  - 20 weeks: Fundus is at umbilicus.
  - 24 to approximately 36 weeks: Fundal height (cm) measured from the symphysis equals the number of weeks of gestation (if a single pregnancy).
- Weight gain
- Optimal weight gain depends on maternal and fetal factors.
  - First trimester the average total weight gain is 1 to 2 kg
  - Approximately 0.5 kg per week for a woman of normal weight during second and third trimesters

Prepregnancy weight	Recommended weight gain
Normal weight	11.3-15.9 kg (25-35 lb)
Underweight	12.7-18.1 kg (28-40 lb)
Overweight	11.3-19.1 kg (25-42 lb)
Multiple birth	Varies with prepregnancy weight

- Psychological maternal changes
  - *Ambivalence:* occurs early in pregnancy, even with a planned pregnancy
  - *Acceptance:* occurs with the woman's readiness for the experience and her identification with the motherhood role; prolonged nonacceptance of the pregnancy is a warning sign
  - *Emotional lability:* rapid unpredictable changes in mood
- Common diagnostic tests
  - Maternal
    - Urine screen
    - Glucose tolerance test
  - Fetal
    - Quad screen includes alpha fetoprotein, human chorionic gonadotropin (hCG), estriol, inhibin A; for high-risk pregnancy, chromosomal abnormalities and neural tube defects
    - Chorionic villi sampling (CVS) for genetic and chromosomal disorders at 8 to 12 weeks; full bladder required; Rh-negative mother requires RhoGAM (Rh$_o$[D] immune globulin) postprocedure
    - Amniocentesis performed at 16 weeks to determine genetic disorders, at 30 weeks to determine lung maturity; bladder emptied if performed after 20 weeks' gestation; Rh-negative mother requires RhoGAM (WinRho [Canada]) postprocedure
    - Ultrasound—multiple purposes; must have full bladder
    - Nonstress test (NST) via ultrasound transducer records fetal movement and heart rate after 28 weeks; increase in heart rate (reactivity) expected in healthy fetus
    - Biophysical profile: includes NST results, amniotic fluid volume, fetal breathing movements, fetal tone and body movements

A client's suspected pregnancy is confirmed. The client tells the nurse that she also has had one pregnancy that she delivered at 39 weeks; twins that she delivered at 34 weeks; and a single gestation that she delivered at 35 weeks. Using the GTPAL notation, how should the nurse record the client's gravidity and parity?

A. 3-0-3-0-3
B. 3-1-1-1-3
C. 4-1-2-0-4
D. 4-2-1-0-3

HESI Test Question Approach

Positive?		YES	NO
Key Words			
Rephrase			
Rule Out Choices			

A	B	C	D

The nurse is monitoring a client in the first stage of labor. The RN identifies fetal heart rate (FHR) decelerations occurring after the onset of each contraction and a return to the baseline well after the contraction is over. Which action(s) should the nurse take? (Select all that apply.)

A. Discontinue oxytocin infusion.
B. Document as a reassuring finding.
C. Give a bolus of 750 mL D_5LR.
D. Assess uterine activity pattern.
E. Administer maternal oxygen.
F. Assess baseline variability.

HESI Test Question Approach

Positive?		YES	NO
Key Words			
Rephrase			
Rule Out Choices			

A	B	C	D	E	F

True Labor

- Pain in lower back radiating to abdomen
- Regular, rhythmic contractions
- Increased intensity with ambulation
- Progressive cervical dilation and effacement

False Labor

- Discomfort localized to abdomen
- No lower back pain
- Contractions often stop with ambulation or position change.

Labor and Delivery

- Stages of labor
  - *First stage*—stage of dilation and effacement and complete with 100% cervical effacement and complete dilation of cervix (10 cm). Duration is from 8 to 20 hours in the primipara and 5 to 14 hours in the multipara. Includes 3 phases, latent (0 to 3 cm), active (4 to 7 cm), and transition (8 to 10 cm).
  - *Second stage*—stage of expulsion and ends with birth of the baby. Generally lasts from a few minutes to 2 hours.

— *Third stage*—the placental separation stage. It begins with the birth of the baby and ends with the expulsion of the placenta. This process can last up to 30 minutes, with an average length of 5 to 10 minutes
— *Fourth stage*—arbitrarily lasts up to 2 hours after delivery of placenta. Monitor for excessive bleeding.

Labor Progression

- *Cervical dilation:* stretching of the cervical os from fingertip diameter to large enough to allow passage of the infant (10 cm)
- *Effacement:* thinning and shortening of the cervix (0% to 100%)
- *Station:* Location of the presenting part in relation to the midpelvis or ischial spines, measured in centimeters above and below, from –5 to +5
  — Station 0 = engaged
  — Station +2 = 2 cm below the level of the ischial spines
  — +5 = crowning
- *Fetal presentation:* part of the fetus that presents to the inlet
- *Position:* relationship of the point of reference (occiput sacrum, acromion) on the fetal presenting part to the mother's pelvis
  — Left occiput anterior (LOA)—most common
- *Lie:* relationship of the long axis (spine) of the fetus to the long axis (spine) of the mother
  — Longitudinal: up and down
  — Transverse: perpendicular
  — Oblique: slanted
- *Attitude:* relationship of fetal parts to one another
  — Flexion: desired, so that smallest diameter of the fetal head is presented
  — Extension can cause dystocia

Nursing and Collaborative Management During Labor

- Assessment
  — Baseline maternal vital signs including pain
  — Medication history
  — Physical assessment
    • Nutrient and fluid intake—hydration and bladder status, need for catheterization, intravenous (IV) therapy
    • Bowel elimination
    • Ambulation and positioning—upright, sitting, squatting best
    • Labs and diagnostic tests
  — Emotional and cultural responses
  — Labor assessment
    • Onset of labor and progression
    • Vaginal exam (assess dilation, effacement, station, position and fetal presentation; omitted in the presence of placenta previa)
    • Status of membranes

- Show
- FHR pattern

— Complications: infection, pregnancy-induced hypertension (PIH), bleeding, prolapsed cord, fetal distress

■ Assessment of contractions (uterine activity pattern)
  — *Duration:* amount of time a contraction lasts, from the beginning to the end
  — *Intensity:* internal monitoring from 30 mm Hg (mild) to 70 mm Hg (strong)
  — *Resting tone/time:* tension of uterine muscle between contractions and time between contractions
  — Characteristics of the FHR
    - Normal range: 110 to 160 beats/min
    - Tachycardia: >160 beats/min
    - Bradycardia: <110 beats/min
    - Variability: change in the heart rate from beat to beat (short term) and cyclic changes over time (long term), in 3 to 5 cycles per minute; moderate long-term variability is reassuring
  — Periodic changes
    - Accelerations—FHR increases with movement; reassuring
    - Decelerations
      □ Early decelerations (reassuring) often occur during second stage and indicate head compression.
      □ Late decelerations (nonreassuring), even if not very "deep," indicate placental insufficiency or hypoxia.
      □ Variable decelerations (nonreassuring), unassociated with contractions, indicate compression of umbilical cord.
      □ The deceleration pattern indicates the insult to the fetus; the variability indicates how well the fetus is tolerating the insult.

Veal Chop Memory Tool

V	Variable decelerations	C	Cord compression
E	Early decelerations	H	Head compression
A	Accelerations	O	OK
L	Late decelerations	P	Placental insufficiency (hypoxia)

External fetal monitoring is noninvasive and is performed with a Toco transducer to measure uterine activity and a Doppler ultrasonic transducer to measure FHR.

Internal fetal monitoring is invasive and requires rupturing of the membranes and attachment of an electrode to the presenting part of the fetus to monitor FHR.

An intrauterine pressure catheter can provide more accurate assessment of uterine tone when needed (use of Pitocin, placental abruption).

During the second stage labor, the nurse notes a pattern of fetal heart rate (FHR) decelerations between 80 and 100 from a baseline of 160. The decelerations are unrelated to the contractions, and moderate long-term baseline FHR variability is present. Place the interventions for these findings in order, starting with the highest priority first.
A. Administer oxygen.
B. Change maternal position.
C. Document the finding.
D. Notify the primary care provider.

HESI Test Question Approach			
Positive?		YES	NO
Key Words			
Rephrase			
Rule Out Choices			
A	B	C	D

A woman who is in labor becomes nauseated, starts hiccupping, and tells her partner to leave her alone. The partner asks the nurse what he did to make this happen. How should the nurse respond?
A. "In active labor, it is quite common for women to react this way. It's nothing you did."
B. "I don't know what you did, but stop, because she is quite sensitive right now."
C. "I'll come and examine her. This reaction is common during the transition phase of labor."
D. "Early labor can be very frustrating. I'm sure she doesn't mean to take it out on you."

HESI Test Question Approach			
Positive?		YES	NO
Key Words			
Rephrase			
Rule Out Choices			
A	B	C	D

The nurse performs a vaginal examination for a laboring client. The RN determines that the cervix is dilated 4 cm with 60% effacement, and the presenting part is at the −2 station. Thirty minutes later, the client calls the RN and says, "I think my water just broke." Which action has the highest priority?
A. Call in the results to the healthcare provider.
B. Evaluate the fetal heart rate.
C. Help the client to the bathroom for hygiene.
D. Perform the nitrazine and fern tests.

HESI Test Question Approach			
Positive?		YES	NO
Key Words			
Rephrase			
Rule Out Choices			
A	B	C	D

Management of Discomfort
Types of Regional Blocks
- Epidural regional anesthesia: peridural (epidural or caudal)
  — Given in first or second stage
  — Single dose or continuously
  — Effective for cesarian delivery
  — Fluid bolus needed to help prevent hypotension

— May prolong second stage

— Increases risk of urinary retention and need for catheter

- Spinal anesthesia (block): intradural (subarachnoid, spinal)—used for cesarian delivery
- Rapid onset
- Client remains flat for 6 to 8 hours after delivery to prevent spinal headache.

Administration of Analgesic Medication

Drugs Used During Labor

- Narcotics—inhibit contractions if given before well-established labor; can cause respiratory depression if given to close to birth; antidote is naloxone (Narcan)
  — Fentanyl
  — Morphine sulfate
  — Hydromorphone (Dilaudid)
- Mixed agonist/antagonists
  — Butorphanol tartrate (Apo-butorphanol [Canada]; Stadol)
  — Nalbuphine (Nubain)

Postpartum Care

Postpartum Maternal Physical Assessment Summary

Memory tool—BUBBLE HA

- Breasts
  — Assess consistency (soft, firm, filling, engorged), nipples (intact, sore, flat, everted or inverted), masses
- Uterus—fundal involution
  — Immediately after delivery: fundus is several centimeters below umbilicus
  — Within 12 hours: fundus rises to umbilicus
  — Descends 1 cm (fingerbreadth) a day for 9 to 10 days; then fundus is below symphysis pubis
  — Should be in midline and firm
- Bladder
  — Measure output; assess for distention or retention.
- Bowel
  — Assess for distention, passing flatus, and bowel sounds.
- Lochia
  — Endometrial sloughing from rubra to serosa to alba
  — Assess color, odor, volume.
- Leg assessment
  — Assess for signs of thrombosis.
- Episiotomy
  — Assess episiotomy or laceration repair for intactness, hematoma, edema, bruising, redness, and drainage.
- Hemorrhoids
  — Sitz bath, Tucks pads, ointments
- Attachment
  — Assess maternal-infant interaction for bonding behaviors

Planning for Discharge

All health plans are required to allow the new mother and newborn to remain in the hospital for a minimum of

48 hours after a normal vaginal birth and for 96 hours after a cesarean birth unless the attending provider, in consultation with the mother, decides on early discharge

Teaching Points

Focus on signs of physical and psychoemotional symptoms of potential problems for mother and infant and how to obtain help.

- Change pads as needed and with voiding/defecation.
- Wipe front to back.
- Good hand-washing technique
- Ice packs, sitz baths, peri-bottle lavage, and topical anesthetic spray and pads
- Breastfeeding instructions
- Balanced diet and adequate fluid intake
- Rest/nap when baby sleeps.
- Contraceptive use and postpartum sexuality
- Postpartum emotions: baby blues, postpartum depression
- Baby care
  — Diapering, bathing, skin and cord care
  — Circumcised or uncircumcised care
  — Newborn behaviors including sleeping habits
  — Jaundice
  — Burping, bowel movements, and wet diapers
- $Rho(D)$ immune globulin (WinRho [Canada]; RhoGAM)
  — Given to Rh-negative women with possible exposure to Rh-positive blood
  — Should have negative indirect Coombs test
  — Given intramuscularly within 72 hours after delivery
  — Checked by two nurses (blood product)
- Rubella vaccine
  — Given subcutaneously to nonimmune client before discharge from hospital
  — May breastfeed
  — Do not give if client or family member is immunocompromised.
  — Avoid pregnancy for 2 to 3 months (teach contraception).

A client who is 72 hours post cesarean delivery is preparing to go home. She shares that she cannot get the baby's diaper on "right." Which action should the nurse take?
A. Demonstrate how to diaper the baby correctly.
B. Observe the client diapering the baby while offering praise and hints.
C. Call the social worker for long-term follow-up.
D. Reassure the client that she knows how to take care of her baby.

HESI Test Question Approach			
Positive?		**YES**	**NO**
Key Words			
Rephrase			
Rule Out Choices			
A	**B**	**C**	**D**

Four births will occur at once. Which birth should the nursery charge nurse assign to a newly licensed nurse as her first solo birth and admission?

A. G1 P0 at 39 weeks who will give birth vaginally after a 15-hour induced labor. The mother has been on magnesium sulfate for pre-eclampsia throughout labor.

B. G5 P4 at 38 weeks who will give birth vaginally after a 5-hour unmedicated labor. Mild to moderate variable decelerations have been occurring for the past 15 minutes.

C. G3 P1 at 34 weeks who will give birth by cesarean delivery for a nonreassuring fetal heart rate pattern. The client has a history of cocaine use and has symptoms of abruptio placentae.

D. G2 P1 at 42 weeks who will give birth vaginally after induced labor. The client has been pushing for 2 hours, and forceps will be used.

Complications of Childbearing

Chronic Hypertension

- Hypertension and/or proteinuria in pregnant woman with chronic hypertension before 20 weeks of gestation and persistent after 12 weeks postpartum

A client at 33 weeks' gestation who has been diagnosed with pregnancy-induced hypertension (PIH) is admitted to the labor and delivery area. She is obviously nervous and expresses concern for the health of her baby. How should the nurse respond?

A. "You have the best doctor on the staff, so don't worry about a thing."

B. "Your anxiety is contributing to your condition and may be the reason for your admission."

C. "This is a minor problem that is easily controlled, and everything will be all right."

D. "As I assess you and your baby, I will explain the plan for your care and answer your questions."

Superimposed Preeclampsia or Eclampsia

- Development of preeclampsia or eclampsia in woman with chronic hypertension before 20 weeks of gestation

Preeclampsia/Eclampsia

HELLP syndrome: life-threatening pregnancy complication usually considered to be a variant of preeclampsia. Can be associated with gestational hypertension: **H**emolysis, **E**levated **L**iver Enzymes, **L**ow **P**latelets—diagnosis made based purely on laboratory values.

- Preeclampsia symptoms
  — Blood pressure
    - Mild: 30 mm Hg systolic and/or 15 mm Hg diastolic over baseline
    - Severe: same (some sources say 160/110 mm Hg × 2 or more)
  — Protein
    - Mild: >1+
    - Severe: 3+ to 4+

HESI Test Question Approach			
Positive?		YES	NO
Key Words			
Rephrase			
Rule Out Choices			
A	B	C	D

HESI Test Question Approach			
Positive?		YES	NO
Key Words			
Rephrase			
Rule Out Choices			
A	B	C	D

— Edema
  - Mild: eyes, face, fingers
  - Severe: generalized edema
— Deep tendon reflexes (DTRs)
  - Mild: may be normal
  - Severe: 3+ or more and clonus
— Central nervous system (CNS) symptoms
  - Mild: headache, irritability
  - Severe: severe headache, visual disturbances
— Other
  - Weight gain >2 lb/week
  - Oliguria (<100 mL/4 hr); epigastric pain related to liver enlargement
  - Elevated serum creatinine, thrombocytopenia, marked SGOT (serum glutamic-oxaloacetic transaminase) elevation

Nursing Interventions: Preeclampsia

- Decrease stimulation in room.
- Explain procedures.
- Maintain IV (16- to 18-g venocatheter).
- Monitor blood pressure every 15 to 30 minutes and DTRs and urine for protein every 1 hour.
- Administer magnesium sulfate as prescribed.
- Monitor magnesium levels and for signs of toxicity (urinary output <30 mL/hr, respiration <12 breaths/min, DTRs absent, deceleration of FHR, bradycardia).

Nursing Interventions: Eclampsia (Seizures)

- Stay with client.
- Turn client on her side.
- Do not attempt to force objects into client's mouth.
- Administer O_2 and have suction available.
- Give magnesium sulfate as prescribed.
- Remember that seizures can occur post partum.
- Magnesium sulfate is not an antihypertensive; it is used to prevent/control seizures. Withhold if any of the following is present:
  — Respiration <12 breaths/min
  — Absent deep tendon reflexes (DTRs)
  — Urine output <30 mL/hr
- Ensure that calcium gluconate 1 g (10 mL of 10% solution) is available for emergency administration to reverse magnesium sulfate toxicity.

Gestational Diabetes

Screening

- Recommendations for glucose screening for all pregnant women
  — 1-hour glucose screen between 24 and 26 weeks
  — Goal is strict blood glucose control.
  — Oral glucose-lowering agents and insulin
    - Generally, glyburide or insulin is used during pregnancy; insulin does not cross the placenta, and glyburide only minimally crosses it.
    - Only regular insulin is used during labor because it is short acting, which makes it easier to maintain the mother's glucose level at 3.3 to 5.6 mmol/L (60 to 100 mg/dL).

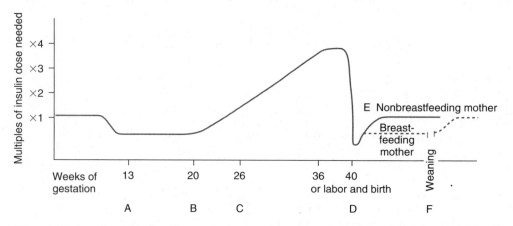

Figure 10-1 Changing insulin needs during pregnancy. (From Lowdermilk D, Perry S, Cashion K, Alden KR: *Maternity and women's health care*, ed 10, St Louis, 2012, Mosby.)

A client who has gestational diabetes asks the nurse to explain why her baby is at risk for macrosomia. Which explanation should the nurse offer?

A. The placenta receives decreased maternal blood flow during pregnancy because of vascular constriction.

B. The fetus secretes insulin in response to maternal hyperglycemia, causing weight gain and growth.

C. Infants of diabetic mothers are postmature, which allows the fetus extra time to grow.

D. Rapid fetal growth contributes to congenital anomalies, which are more common in infants of diabetic mothers.

HESI Test Question Approach			
Positive?		**YES**	**NO**
Key Words			
Rephrase			
Rule Out Choices			
A	**B**	**C**	**D**

Preterm Labor (PTL)

- Signs and symptoms of PTL
  — More than five contractions in an hour
  — Menstrual-like cramps
  — Low, dull backache
  — Pelvic pressure
  — Increase/change in vaginal discharge
  — Leaking or gush of amniotic fluid

Tocolytics and Their Administration

Tocolytics stop uterine contractions.

- Ritodrine (Yutopar)
  — Side effects
    • Nervousness and tremulousness
    • Headache
    • Nausea/vomiting, diarrhea, epigastric pain
  — Adverse effects
    • Tachycardia
    • Chest pain with pulmonary edema
    • Low K$^+$, hyperglycemia
  — Nursing interventions
    • Maternal electrocardiogram (ECG) and laboratory tests

- Cardiac and fetal monitoring
- Vital signs every 15 minutes
— Antidote
— Propranolol (Inderal)
- Terbutaline (Brethine)
— Side effects
  - Nervousness and tremulousness
  - Headache
  - Nausea/vomiting, diarrhea, epigastric pain
— Adverse effects
  - Tachycardia
  - Chest pain with pulmonary edema
  - Low K^+, hyperglycemia
— Nursing interventions
  - Notify health care provider if the woman exhibits the following:
    - Maternal heart rate greater than 130 beats/min; arrhythmias, chest pain
    - Blood pressure <90/60 mm Hg
    - Signs of pulmonary edema (e.g., dyspnea, crackles, decreased Sao_2)
    - Fetal heart rate >180 beats/min
  - Hyperglycemia occurs more frequently in women who are being treated simultaneously with corticosteroids.
  - Ensure that the antidote propranolol (Inderal) is available to reverse adverse effects related to cardiovascular function.
  - Monitor intake and output.
  - Check weight daily.
- Magnesium sulfate
— Side effects
  - CNS depression
  - Slowed respirations
  - Decreased DTRs
— Adverse effects
  - Decreased urine output
  - Pulmonary edema
— Nursing interventions
  - Hold if:
    - Respirations <12 breaths/min
    - Urine output <100 mL/4 hr
    - Absent DTRs
— Monitor serum magnesium levels with higher doses; therapeutic range is between 4 and 7.5 mEq/L or 5 and 8 mg/dL.
— Antidote
  - Ensure that calcium gluconate 1 g (10 mL of 10% solution) is available for emergency administration to reverse magnesium sulfate toxicity.
- Drugs used to decrease contractions
— Indomethacin (Indocin)
— Calcium channel blocker—nifedipine (Procardia)
— Nitroglycerin
- Betamethasone (Celestone) is used in PTL to enhance surfactant production and fetal lung maturity if the fetus is <35 weeks' gestation.

A client at 15 weeks' gestation is admitted for an inevitable abortion. Thirty minutes after returning from surgery, her vital signs are stable. Which nursing intervention has the highest priority?

A. Ask the client if she would like to talk about losing her baby.
B. Place cold cabbage leaves on the client's breasts to reduce breast engorgement.
C. Send a referral to the grief counselor for at-home follow-up.
D. Confirm the client's Rh and Coombs status and administer RhoGAM (WinRho) if indicated.

HESI Test Question Approach			
Positive?		YES	NO
Key Words			
Rephrase			
Rule Out Choices			
A	B	C	D

Spontaneous Abortion

Nursing Assessment

- Vaginal bleeding with a gestational age of 20 weeks or less
- Uterine cramping, backache, and pelvic pressure
- May have symptoms of shock
- Assess client/family emotional status and needs, and provide support.

Nursing and Collaborative Management

- Monitor vital signs, level of consciousness, and amount of bleeding.
- Prepare client to receive IV fluids and/or blood.
- If client is Rh negative, give RhoGAM (WinRho).

Incompetent Cervix

Incompetent cervix (recurrent premature dilation of the cervix) is passive, painless dilation of the cervix during the second trimester.

- Conservative management
  - Bed rest
  - Hydration
  - Tocolysis (inhibition of uterine contractions)
- Cervical cerclage may be performed.
  - McDonald cerclage: band of homologous fascia or nonabsorbable ribbon (Mersilene) may be placed around the cervix beneath the mucosa to constrict the internal os of the cervix
  - Cerclage procedure can be classified according to time or whether it is elective (prophylactic), urgent, or emergent.

Ectopic Pregnancy

Nursing Assessment

- Missed period but early signs of pregnancy absent
- Positive pregnancy test result
- Rupture
  - Sharp, unilateral pelvic pain
  - Vaginal bleeding
  - Referred shoulder pain
  - Syncope can lead to shock.

Nursing and Collaborative Management

- Monitor hemodynamic status.
- Prepare client for surgery and IV fluid administration, including blood.

Abruptio Placentae and Placenta Previa

Abruptio Placentae

— Concealed or overt bleeding
— Uterine tone ranges from tense without relaxation to tense and board like.
— Persistently painful
— Abnormal fetal heart rate—nonreassuring fetal heart rate pattern (the more area abrupted, the worse the FHR)

Placenta Previa

— Bright red vaginal bleeding
— Soft uterine tone
— Painless
— FHR is normal unless bleeding is severe and mother becomes hypovolemic.

- If abruption or previa is suspected or confirmed, no abdominal or vaginal manipulation such as
  — Leopold's maneuvers
  — Vaginal examinations
  — Internal monitor (especially if previa)
  — Rectal examinations/enemas/suppositories

Disseminated Intravascular Coagulation

- Risk factors for DIC in pregnancy
  — Fetal demise
  — Infection/sepsis
  — Pregnancy-induced hypertension (pre-eclampsia)
  — Abruptio placentae

Dystocia

- A difficult birth resulting from problems involving the 5Ps (powers, passage, passenger, psyche, and/or position); a lack of progress in cervical dilation, delay in fetal descent, or change in uterine contraction characteristics suggests dystocia.

Postpartum Complications

- Hemorrhage
  — Assess fundal location and consistency
  — Assess vaginal bleeding; saturating pad per hour indicates hemorrhage
  — Monitor for signs of shock.
  — Assess for bladder distention; can prevent involution and lead to hemorrhage
- Venous thromboembolism
  — Related to venous stasis and hypercoagulability
  — Can result in superficial venous thrombosis, deep vein thrombosis, or pulmonary embolism
  — Assess legs for pain, tenderness, swelling.
  — Treated with bed rest, anticoagulants, leg elevation, analgesia

- Infection
  — Perineal infections
  — Endometritis
  — Parametritis
  — Peritonitis
  — Mastitis
  — Cystitis
  — Pyelonephritis
- HIV, hepatitis, other sexually transmitted diseases
- Postpartum depression
  — Blues—emotionally labile from 5 to 10 days post partum; reinforce need to rest, obtain support from family friends and community
  — Depression—occurs within 4 weeks of childbirth; irritability ruminations of guilt and inadequacy; may have rejection of the infant; supportive treatment including antidepressant agents and psychotherapy

The nurse receives shift reports on four postpartum clients. Which client should the nurse assess first?
A. G3 P3, 7 hours after forceps delivery, who complains of pain and perineal pressure unrelieved by analgesics
B. G1 P1, 8 hours after cesarean delivery, who is receiving IV oxytocin (Pitocin) and complains of cramping with increased lochia when sitting
C. G2 P2, 5 hours after vaginal delivery, who complains of abdominal pain when the infant breastfeeds
D. G7 P6, 6 hours after vaginal delivery of twins, who reports saturating one pad in a 3-hour period

Which nursing action has the highest priority for an infant immediately after birth?
A. Place the infant's head in the "sniff" position and give oxygen via face mask.
B. Perform a bedside glucose test and feed the infant glucose water as needed.
C. Assess the heart rate and perform chest compressions if the heart rate is less than 60 beats/min.
D. Dry the newborn and place the infant under a radiant warmer or skin-to-skin with the mother.

Newborn Parameters (Approximate)

- Length: 18 to 22 inches
- Weight: 5.5 to 9.5 lb
- Head circumference: 13.2 to 14 inches
- Head should be one fourth the body length
- Sutures are palpable with fontanels
- Fontanel closure
  — Anterior: by 18 months
  — Posterior: 6 to 8 weeks

HESI Test Question Approach			
Positive?		YES	NO
Key Words			
Rephrase			
Rule Out Choices			
A	B	C	D

HESI Test Question Approach			
Positive?		YES	NO
Key Words			
Rephrase			
Rule Out Choices			
A	B	C	D

- Umbilical cord should have three vessels: two arteries and one vein
- Extremities should be flexed.
- Major gluteal folds even
- Creases on soles of feet
- Ortolani's sign and Barlow's sign for developmental dysplasia of the hip
- Pulses palpable (radial, brachial, femoral)

Newborn Vital Signs

- Heart rate (resting): 100 to 160 beats/min (apical) by auscultating at the fourth intercostal space for 1 full minute
- Respirations: 30 to 60 breaths/min for 1 full minute
- Axillary temperature: 36° to 37.2 °C (96.8° to 99 °F)
- Blood pressure: 73/55 mm Hg

Hypoglycemia

- Assess for risk factors in maternal history (infant of the diabetic mother) and environmental factors (cold stress)
- Parameters are for full-term infants
  - Low blood glucose level
    - <1.7 mmol/L (30 mg/dL) in the first 72 hours of life
    - <2.5 mmol/L (35 mg/dL) after the first 3 days of life
  - Normal blood glucose level
    - 1.7 to 3.3 mmol/L (30 to 60 mg/dL) in 1-day-old newborn
    - 2.2 to 5.0 mmol/L (40 to 90 mg/dL) in newborn >1 day

Nursing and Collaborative Management

- Keep newborn warm.
- Suction airway as necessary.
- Observe for respiratory distress.
- Normal or physiological jaundice appears after the first 24 hours in full-term newborns.
- Pathological jaundice occurs before this time and may indicate early hemolysis of red blood cells.
- Assess hemoglobin and hematocrit and blood glucose levels.
- Weigh daily.
- Monitor intake and output; weigh diapers if necessary (1 g = 1 mL of urine).
- Monitor temperature.
- Observe for any cracks in the skin.
- Administer eye medication within 1 hour after birth.
- Provide cord care.
- Provide circumcision care and teach mother how to care for circumcision site.
- Position newborn on right side after feeding; however, the side-lying position is not recommended for sleep because this position makes it easy for the newborn to roll to the prone position.
- Observe for normal stool and passage of meconium.
- Test newborn's reflexes.

Reflexes Exhibited and Age Reflexes Disappear

- Sucking or rooting: 3 to 4 months
- Moro reflex: 3 to 4 months
- Tonic neck or fencing: 3 to 4 months
- Babinski's sign: 1 year to 18 months
- Palmar-plantar grasp: 8 months
- Stepping or walking: 3 to 4 months

Major Newborn Complications

Respiratory Distress Syndrome

- Caused by immaturity of lungs and inability to produce surfactant
- Results in hypoxia and acidosis

Meconium Aspiration Syndrome

- Can be a sign of fetal distress, which increases intestinal peristalsis
- Fetus or newborn aspirates meconium-stained fluid, thick meconium indicates higher risk.
- Meconium staining more common in breech presentation, postterm deliveries

Retinopathy of Prematurity

- Damage to retinal vessels caused by the prolonged use of oxygen (>30 days)
- Infants receiving oxygen therapy examined by ophthalmologist

Hyperbilirubinemia

- Jaundice becomes visible when the total serum bilirubin (TSB) reaches 85 mcmol/L (5 to 6 mg/dL). Jaundice is considered abnormal or nonphysiologic when TSB rises more rapidly and to higher levels than is expected or stays elevated for longer than normal.
- Prevention of kernicterus, which results in permanent neurological damage
- Jaundice starts at head, spreads to chest, abdomen, arms, legs, hands, and feet
- Phototherapy: use of fluorescent light to reduce serum bilirubin levels (phototherapy blankets eliminate the hazards of overhead light therapy)
- Possible adverse effects: eye damage, dehydration, sensory deprivation
- Expose as much of the skin as possible but cover genital area.
- Cover the eyes with eye shields.
- Monitor skin temperature closely.
- Increase fluids to compensate for water loss.
- Expect loose green stools and green urine.
- Monitor newborn's skin color.
- Reposition every 2 hours.
- Provide stimulation.
- After treatment, continue monitoring for signs of rebound hyperbilirubinemia.

Erythroblastosis Fetalis

- Destruction of red blood cells as a result of an antigen-antibody reaction

- Characterized by hemolytic anemia or hyperbilirubinemia
- Exchange of fetal and maternal blood occurs at birth; antibodies are harmless to the mother but cause fetal hemolysis.
- Administer Rho(D) immune globulin (WinRho).
- Newborn's blood is replaced with Rh-negative blood to stop destruction of newborn's red blood cells.
- Rh-negative blood gradually is replaced with newborn's own blood.

Sepsis
- Presence of bacteria in the blood
- Prevention—antibiotics in labor for group B *Streptococcus* positive
- Assess for maternal, intrapartum, and neonatal risk factors.
- Early signs are nonspecific and include lethargy, poor feeding, poor weight gain, and irritability.

TORCH Infections
- Infections involving one of the following:
  — **T**oxoplasmosis
  — **O**ther infections (e.g., gonorrhea, syphilis, varicella, hepatitis B, HIV, or human parvovirus B19)
  — **R**ubella
  — **C**ytomegalovirus
  — **H**erpes simplex virus

Substance Abuse
- Effects on fetus vary according to substance
- Narcotics cause passive addiction: neonatal abstinence syndrome
- Treatment of drug-exposed newborns focuses on reduction of external stimuli, supportive treatment of symptoms, and sedation.
- Fetal alcohol syndrome
  — Caused by maternal alcohol use during pregnancy
  — Associated with neurological problems, IQ deficit, and attention-deficit/hyperactivity disorder
  — Craniofacial features include microcephaly, small eyes or short palpebral fissures, a thin upper lip, a flat midface, and an indistinct philtrum.

Newborn of a Mother with HIV
- Monitor antibody closely throughout pregnancy.
- Testing and treatment in pregnancy greatly reduce risk of transmission to fetus.

Infant of a Mother with Diabetes
- Infant born to mother with type 1 or type 2 diabetes or gestational diabetes
- Newborn may have hypoglycemia, hypocalcemia, hypomagnesemia, polycythemia, hyperbilirubinemia, cardiomyopathy, respiratory distress syndrome (RDS), birth trauma, and congenital anomalies.

A pregnant client tells the nurse that she smokes only a few cigarettes a day. What information should the nurse provide the client about the effects of smoking during pregnancy?

A. Smoking causes vasoconstriction and reduces placental perfusion.

B. Smoking reduces the lecithin:sphingomyelin ratio, contributing to lung immaturity.

C. Smoking causes vasodilation and increased fluid overload for the fetus.

D. Smoking during pregnancy places the fetus at risk for lung cancer.

HESI Test Question Approach			
Positive?		YES	NO
Key Words			
Rephrase			
Rule Out Choices			
A	B	C	D

11 Mental Health Nursing

Nurse-Client Relationship

- The goal of the nurse-client relationship is to facilitate quality client-centered care by using verbal and nonverbal communication to build trust, provide comfort, and encourage change.
- Privacy and confidentiality: a client's reasonable expectation that information revealed to the nurse will not be disclosed to others. However, the nurse must explain to the client that information relevant to the individual's treatment plan must be shared with the other members of the treatment team, especially if the client has thoughts of harming himself or herself or others.

Therapeutic Communication

- Both verbal and nonverbal expression
- Goal directed
- Appropriate, efficient, flexible, and elicits feedback
- Basic communication principles can be applied to all clients:
  — Establish trust.
  — Demonstrate a nonjudgmental attitude
  — Offer self; be empathetic, not sympathetic.
  — Use active listening.
  — Accept and support client's feelings.
  — Clarify and validate client's statements.
  — Use a matter-of-fact approach.
- Examples of therapeutic communication
  — Silence: sit quietly and wait; silence is planned.
  — Active listening: gives full attention to the client
  — Open-ended questioning: promotes sharing
  — Empathizing: demonstrating warmth and acknowledgment of feelings
  — Restating: repeats what the client says to show understanding and to review what was said.

Mental Health

- Mental health is a lifelong process of adjustment to changing environments (internal and external).

Mental Health Illness

Mental health illness is the loss of the ability to respond to the environment in accord with oneself and society. In many clients it is a temporary loss.

An adult client is admitted to the in-client mental health unit for severe depression. Although the client has agreed to electroconvulsive therapy (ECT), the client's partner states, "I'm concerned that his neurons will be destroyed by this treatment." Which response by the nurse is most helpful?

A. "I'll contact the nurse supervisor for you."
B. "Let's tour the ECT room and speak to the staff."
C. "I think you should show support for your partner."
D. "May we sit and discuss your concerns about ECT?"

HESI Test Question Approach			
Positive?		YES	NO
Key Words			
Rephrase			
Rule Out Choices			
A	B	C	D

A female client who has just learned that she has breast cancer tells her family that the biopsy was negative. What action should the nurse take?

A. Remind the client that the results were positive.
B. Ask the client to restate what the healthcare provider told her.
C. Talk to the family about the client's need for family support.
D. Encourage the client to talk to the nurse about her fears.

HESI Test Question Approach			
Positive?		YES	NO
Key Words			
Rephrase			
Rule Out Choices			
A	B	C	D

Coping and Defense Mechanisms

- Primarily unconscious efforts to reduce anxiety
- Can be constructive or destructive
- *Coping* is related to problem solving
- *Defense* is related to protecting oneself
  — *Examples:* denial, displacement, identification

Treatment Modalities

- *Milieu therapy:* takes place in the physical and social environment in which the client is receiving treatment
- *Interpersonal psychotherapy:* uses a therapeutic relationship to modify the client's feelings, attitudes, and behaviors
- *Behavior therapy:* takes many forms and is used to change the client's behaviors
- *Cognitive therapy:* directive, time-limited approach
- *Crisis intervention:* directed at resolution of the immediate crisis and to returning the individual to the precrisis level of functioning
- *Electroconvulsive therapy (ECT):* a physical treatment for psychiatric disorders using electrically induced seizures to treat severely depressed individuals who fail to respond to antidepressant medications and therapy

The nurse is facilitating a support group for stress management. During the initial phase, a female group member states that she can help the group more because she has a master's degree. How should the nurse respond?

A. Restate the purpose of the support group sessions.
B. Ask the group to identify various stressful problems.
C. Obtain ideas from the members about strategies for stressful situations.
D. Conclude the meeting and evaluate the session.

HESI Test Question Approach			
Positive?		**YES**	**NO**
Key Words			
Rephrase			
Rule Out Choices			
A	**B**	**C**	**D**

Group Therapy

- Involves a therapist and five to eight members
- Provides feedback and support for the individual goals of each member
- Group therapy models
  — Psychoanalytical
  — Transactional analysis
  — Rogerian therapy
  — Gestalt therapy
- Interpersonal group therapy
- Self-help or support groups
- Family therapy
  — The member with the presenting symptoms indicates the presence of problems in the entire family
  — A change in one member brings about changes in other members
- Therapeutic factors in groups
  — *Instillation of hope and optimism* about group treatment
  — *Universality:* Members realize they are not alone with their problems, feelings, or thoughts.
  — *Imparting of information:* Members receive formal teaching by the leader or advice from peers.
  — *Altruism:* Members feel a reward from giving support to others.
  — *Recapitulation:* Members repeat patterns of behavior in the group that they learned in their families; feedback from the leader and peers provides opportunities to learn about their behavior.
  — *Development of socializing techniques:* Members learn new social skills based on feedback from others.
  — *Imitative behavior:* Members copy behavior from the leaders or peers and can adopt healthier habits.
  — *Interpersonal learning:* Members gain insight into themselves based on feedback from others; occurs later in group after establishing trust.
  — *Group cohesiveness:* In a mature group, members accept positive feedback and constructive criticism.
  — *Catharsis:* Intense feelings, as judged by the member, are shared.
  — *Existential resolution:* Members learn to accept painful aspects of life (i.e., loneliness, death) that affect everyone.

Stages of Group Development

- Initial stage: superficial communication
- Working stage: real work is done by group
- Termination stage: provides opportunity to learn to deal with letting go

The nurse and the unlicensed assistive personnel take a group of mental health clients to a baseball game. During the game, a male client begins to complain of shortness of breath and dizziness. Which intervention should the nurse implement first?

A. Send the client back to the unit.
B. Ask for a description of his feelings.
C. Escort the client to a quiet area.
D. Inquire about what is most stressful.

HESI Test Question Approach			
Positive?		**YES**	**NO**
Key Words			
Rephrase			
Rule Out Choices			
A	**B**	**C**	**D**

Anxiety

Anxiety is a normal subjective experience that includes feelings of apprehension, uneasiness, uncertainty, or dread.

Types of Anxiety

- *Mild:* tension of everyday life
- *Moderate:* immediate concerns
- *Severe:* feeling that something bad is about to happen
- *Panic:* terror and a sense of impending doom

Anxiety Disorders

Generalized Anxiety Disorder

- Unrealistic anxiety about everyday worries
- Panic disorders—produce a sudden feeling of intense apprehension

Phobias

- Irrational fear of an object, activity, or situation
- Client may recognize fear as unreasonable
- Associated with panic-level anxiety
- Defense mechanisms include repression and displacement (i.e., agoraphobia)

Nursing and Collaborative Management

- Reduce stimuli in the environment.
- Provide a calm, quiet environment.
- Administer antianxiety medications as prescribed.
- Administer selective serotonin reuptake inhibitors (SSRIs) and tricyclic antidepressants (TCAs) as prescribed.

The nurse is planning to teach a male client strategies for coping with his anxiety. The nurse finds him in his room, compulsively washing his hands. What action should the nurse take next?

A. Teach him alternatives as he washes his hands.
B. Ask him to stop his hand washing immediately.
C. Allow him to finish hand washing before teaching.
D. Ask what precipitated the hand washing.

HESI Test Question Approach			
Positive?		YES	NO
Key Words			
Rephrase			
Rule Out Choices			
A	B	C	D

Obsessive-Compulsive Disorder

- *Obsessions:* persistently intrusive thoughts
- *Compulsions:* repetitive behaviors designed to divert unacceptable thought and reduce anxiety (i.e., hoarding disorder)

Antianxiety (Anxiolytic) Medications

- These drugs depress the central nervous system.
  - **Benzodiazepines** have anxiety-reducing (anxiolytic), sedative-hypnotic, muscle-relaxing, and anticonvulsant actions.
  - **Flumazenil** (Anexate [Canada]; Romazicon), a benzodiazepine antagonist administered intravenously, reverses benzodiazepine intoxication in 5 minutes.

Somatic Symptom Disorder

Persistent worry or complaints about physical illness without physical findings.

- Types of somatoform disorders
  - Conversion disorder (functional neurological)
  - Hypochondriasis
  - Somatization disorders
  - Factitious disorder
- Treatment: cognitive behavioral therapy

The nurse is talking to a client with a dissociative identity disorder. During the interaction, the client begins to dissociate. Which action should the nurse take?

A. Escort the client to art therapy group.
B. Call the client by name.
C. Talk about stressful feelings.
D. Move to another setting.

HESI Test Question Approach			
Positive?		YES	NO
Key Words			
Rephrase			
Rule Out Choices			
A	B	C	D

Crisis Intervention

- A crisis results from the experiencing of a significant traumatic event or situation that cannot be remedied by the use of available coping strategies.
- Risk factors include multiple comorbidities, multiple losses, unexpected life changes, limited coping skills, chronic pain or disability, poor social support, concurrent psychiatric disorders, substance abuse or disability, and limited access to healthcare service.
- Goal is to return client to precrisis level of functioning

Nursing and Collaborative Management

- Assess for suicidal or homicidal thoughts or plans.
- Help client feel safe and less anxious.
- Listen carefully.
- Be directive (e.g., nurse may arrange for shelter or contact a social worker).
- Mobilize social support.
- Involve client in identifying realistic, acceptable interventions.
- Plan regular follow-up.

Trauma-Stressor-Related Disorders

Acute Stress

- Abnormal response to an extreme abnormal event (witnessing a horrific car accident or war-zone blast)

Acute Stress Disorder

- Occurs within a month of an individual who experiences or sees an event involving death, severe injury, or physical violation to the individual or others

Posttraumatic Stress Disorder

- Reexperience of traumatic event involving (or real threat of) death, serious injury, or physical violation
- Recurrent and intrusive dreams or flashbacks

Dissociative Disorders

These disorders are associated with exposure to an extremely traumatic event.

- *Dissociative amnesia:* one or more episodes of inability to recall important personal information, usually of a traumatic nature
- *Dissociative identity disorder:* two or more distinct identities, at least two of which recurrently take control
- *Depersonalization/derealization disorder:* persistent or recurrent episodes of feelings of detachment from oneself

Personality Disorders

- Inflexible maladaptive behavior patterns
- In touch with reality
- Lack of insight into one's behavior

- Forms of acting out (often seen in clients with border-line personality disorder)
  — Yelling and swearing
  — Cutting oneself
  — Manipulation
  — Substance abuse
  — Promiscuous sexual behaviors
  — Suicide attempts

A female client who has borderline personality disorder returns after a weekend pass with lacerations to both wrists. The client complains to the nurse during the dressing change. The tone of the nurse's response should be:
A. Distant
B. Concerned
C. Matter of fact
D. Empathetic

HESI Test Question Approach		
Positive?	**YES**	**NO**
Key Words		
Rephrase		
Rule Out Choices		
A	B	C	D

Eating Disorders

Compulsive Overeating
- Bingelike overeating without purging
- Lack of control over food consumption

Anorexia Nervosa
- Onset often associated with a stressful event
- Death can occur from starvation, suicide, cardiomyopathies, or electrolyte imbalance
- Client experiences a distorted body image

Bulimia Nervosa
- Binge-purge syndrome in which eating binges are followed by purging behaviors

A client with bulimia is admitted to the mental health unit. What intervention is most important for the nurse to include in the initial treatment plan?
A. Observe the client after meals for vomiting.
B. Assess daily weight and vital signs.
C. Monitor serum potassium and calcium.
D. Provide a structured environment at mealtime.

HESI Test Question Approach		
Positive?	**YES**	**NO**
Key Words		
Rephrase		
Rule Out Choices		
A	B	C	D

The mental health RN is assigned to four clients. Which client should be assessed first?

A. A newly admitted client diagnosed with major depression whose assessment is incomplete
B. A client with schizophrenia who is having auditory hallucinations of someone crying
C. A client who recently became unemployed and has a 10-year history of daily alcohol use
D. A client with anorexia nervosa having difficulty attending group therapy

HESI Test Question Approach			
Positive?		**YES**	**NO**
Key Words			
Rephrase			
Rule Out Choices			
A	**B**	**C**	**D**

Depressive Disorders

Major Depressive Disorder

- Dysthymia (persistent depressive disorder)
- Premenstrual dysphoric disorder
- Substance/medication-induced depressive disorder
- Depressive disorder due to another medical condition

Depression

- Characterized by feelings of hopelessness, low self-esteem, self-blame
- Twenty-five percent of those with depression have suicidal ideation
- Behavior therapy, cognitive behavioral therapy, and interpersonal psychotherapy
- Antidepressant medication therapy
  — Cyclic antidepressants (e.g., TCAs)
  — SSRIs and serotonin-norepinephrine reuptake inhibitors (SNRIs)
  — Atypical antidepressants

Suicide

- A suicide threat is a warning, direct or indirect, verbal or nonverbal, that a person is planning to take his or her own life.
- The person may give away prized possessions, make a will or funeral arrangements, or withdraw from friendships and social activities.
- Assessment includes whether the person has made a specific plan and whether the means to carry out the plan are available.
- NEVER leave a suicidal client alone.
- Protect the client from inflicting harm, be vigilant, supervise medication administration, and implement strategies to increase self-esteem and social support.
- Be aware of major warning signs of impending attempt.
  — Client begins to give away possessions.
  — Client becomes "better" or "happy."

Bipolar Disorder

- Bipolar I or II
- Characterized by episodes of mania and/or depression with periods of normal mood and activity in between
- Lithium carbonate is the medication of choice; it can be toxic and requires regular monitoring of serum lithium levels.
- Other medications
  — Divalproex (Depakote, Valproate)
  — Olanzapine (Zyprexa)
  — Carbamazepine (Tegretol)

Purpose of Antidepressants

Antidepressants have been approved for depression, phobias, eating disorders, and anxiety disorders.

Monoamine Oxidase Inhibitors (MAOIs)

- Inhibit the enzyme monoamine oxidase, which is present in the brain, blood platelets, liver, spleen, and kidneys
- Administered to clients with depression who have not responded to other antidepressant therapies, including electroconvulsive therapy
- Concurrent use with amphetamines, antidepressants, dopamine, epinephrine, guanethidine, levodopa, methyldopa, nasal decongestants, norepinephrine, reserpine, tyramine-containing foods, or vasoconstrictors may cause hypertensive crisis.
- Concurrent use with opioid analgesics may cause hypertension or hypotension, coma, or seizures.

Nursing Implications and Client Education

- Selective serotonin reuptake inhibitors (SSRIs)
  — Inhibit serotonin uptake
- Tricyclic antidepressants (TCAs)
  — Block the reuptake of norepinephrine (and serotonin) at the presynaptic neuron
  — May take several weeks to produce the desired effect (2 to 4 weeks after the first dose)
  — NOTE: Trazodone can cause priapism in males and rarely in females [clitoris])

HIGH ALERT Antidepressant Use

- *Serotonin syndrome*
  — Hyperthermia, rigidity, cognitive impairments, and autonomic symptoms
  — Potentially fatal and may occur at any time during therapy with SSRIs combined with MAOIs
  — Treatment is symptomatic with propranolol, cooling blankets, chlorpromazine for hyperthermia, diazepam for muscle rigidity or rigors
- *Antidepressant apathy:* Some clients lose interest in life and the events around them.
- *Antidepressant withdrawal syndrome:* Abrupt cessation of antidepressants engenders withdrawal symptoms.
- *Antidepressant loss of effectiveness:* Sometimes medications are no longer effective.
- *Antidepressant-induced suicide:* especially among 18- to 24-year-olds in the early stages of treatment

Schizophrenia Spectrum and Other Psychotic Disorders

- Schizophrenia, schizoaffective disorder, delusional disorder, and catatonia
- A group of mental disorders characterized by psychotic features
  — Delusions are thought or beliefs.
  - *Delusions of persecution:* Client believes he or she is being persecuted by some powerful force.
  - *Delusions of grandeur:* Client has an exaggerated sense of self that has no basis in reality.
  - *Somatic delusions:* Client believes his or her body is changing, with no basis in reality.
- Perceptual distortions
  — *Illusions:* brief experiences of misinterpretation or misperception of reality that usually occur with delirium, delirium tremens, or drug induced (i.e., a person misperceives a coat hanging in the hall as a threatening animal)
  — *Hallucinations* (five senses): false perceptions with no basis in reality (i.e., hearing voices when no one is speaking)
  — *Safety is the first priority:* Make sure client does not have an auditory command telling him or her to harm himself or herself or others.

Nursing and Collaborative Management

- Assess for risk of violence to self or others and take appropriate precautions.
- Provide quiet, soothing environment.
- Establish routine and boundaries.
- Provide stable, nonthreatening, brief, social interactions.
- If acting frightened or scared, increase physical space surrounding client and approach calmly.
- Encourage reality-based interests.

Antipsychotic Medications

- Traditional medications
- Purpose: treat psychotic behavior
  — Side effects
  - Extrapyramidal syndrome (EPS)
  - Akathisia (e.g., pacing, rocking motions)
  - Acute dystonia (e.g., muscle cramps of head and neck)
  - Pseudoparkinsonism (stiffening of muscular activity in face, body, arms, and legs, cogwheel rigidity)
  - Anticholinergic
  — Nursing implications
  - Screen for EPS using Abnormal Involuntary Movement Scale (AIMS)
  - Encourage fluid (water)
  - Gum
  - Hard candy
  - Increase fiber intake
- Long-acting medications
  — Promote medication compliance
  — Side effects

- Blood dyscrasias
- Neuroleptic malignant syndrome
  — Nursing implications
  - Change position slowly for dizziness
  - Report urinary retention to healthcare provider
- Atypical medications
  — Purpose: treat all positive and negative symptoms
  — Side effects: multiple side effects, depending on medication
  — Nursing implications
  - Tolerance to effects usually occurs.
  - Neuroleptic malignant syndrome (NMS) involving autonomic, motor, and behavioral symptoms: the antipsychotic agent should be stopped immediately if the patient develops signs of NMS such as severe muscle rigidity, confusion, agitation, and increased temperature, pulse, and blood pressure

Substance Abuse Disorders

- *Substance dependence:* a pattern of repeated use of a substance
- *Substance tolerance:* a need for more of the substance to reach the desired effect
- *Substance abuse:* recurrent use of a substance
- *Substance withdrawal:* the occurrence of symptoms when blood levels of a substance decline

Alcohol Abuse
Alcohol is a central nervous system (CNS) depressant.
- *Physical dependence:* a biological need for alcohol to avoid physical withdrawal symptoms
- *Psychological dependence:* a craving for the subjective effect of alcohol
- *Intoxication:* blood alcohol level ≥0.1% (21.7 mmol/L [100 mg alcohol/dL] blood)

Alcohol Withdrawal
- Signs peak after 24 to 48 hours.
- Chlordiazepoxide (Librium) is the "gold standard," the most commonly prescribed medication for acute alcohol withdrawal.
- Withdrawal delirium: peaks 48 to 72 hours after cessation of intake and lasts 2 to 3 days
  — **Medical emergency**
  — Death can occur from myocardial infarction, fat emboli, peripheral vascular collapse, electrolyte imbalance, aspiration pneumonia, or suicide.

Disulfiram (Antabuse) Therapy
- Alcohol deterrent
- Other medications used to assist with cravings
  — Acamprosate calcium (Campral)
  — Naltrexone (ReVia)
- Instruct client taking disulfiram to avoid the use of substances that contain alcohol, such as cough medicines, mouthwashes, and aftershave lotions.

A male client with a history of alcohol abuse is admitted to the medical unit for gastrointestinal bleeding and pancreatitis. His admission data include blood pressure 156/96 mm Hg, pulse 92 beats/min, and temperature 37.3 °C (99.2 °F). Which intervention is most important for the nurse to implement?

A. Provide a quiet, low-stimulus environment.
B. Initiate seizure precautions.
C. Administer as needed (PRN) lorazepam (Ativan) as prescribed.
D. Determine the time and quantity of the client's last alcohol intake.

HESI Test Question Approach			
Positive?		YES	NO
Key Words			
Rephrase			
Rule Out Choices			
A	B	C	D

Neurocognitive Disorders

Autism Spectrum Disorder

- Etiology: no known cause
- Clinical description
  - Hyperactivity
  - Short attention span
  - Impulsivity
  - Aggressivity
  - Self-injurious behavior
  - Temper tantrums
  - Repetitive mannerisms
  - Preoccupied with objects
  - Spoken language often absent
  - "Islands of genius"
- Prognosis: There is no cure for autism. Language skills and intellectual level are the strongest factors related to the prognosis. Only a small percentage of individuals with the disorder go on to live and work independently as adults.
- *Asperger's disorder* has many features similar to those of autism but does not show significant delays in language, cognitive development, age-appropriate self-help skills, adaptive behavior, or curiosity about the environment. It is a lifelong disorder.

Attention-Deficit/Hyperactivity Disorder

- Etiology: no known cause but strong correlation with genetic factors
- Clinical description
  - Fidgeting in a seat
  - Getting up when expected to be seated
  - Excessive running when dangerous or inappropriate
  - Loud, disruptive play during quiet activities
  - Forgets and misses appointments
  - Fails to meet deadlines
  - Loses the train of conversation
  - Changes topics inappropriately
  - Does not follow rules of games

- Prognosis: Condition continues into adolescence in most children; many adults who had ADHD in childhood report a decrease of hyperactivity but a continuation of difficulty concentrating or attending to complex projects.
- Clients with ADHD may require CNS stimulants to reduce hyperactive behavior and lengthen attention span.

Neurocognitive Disorders

Major and mild neurocognitive disorders (NCD) (DSM-5 terminology that includes dementia)

Dementia
- Dementia is a syndrome of progressive deterioration in intellectual functioning secondary to structural or functional changes.
- Marked by long-term and short-term memory loss
- Impairment in judgment, abstract thinking, problem-solving ability, and behavior also seen
- Most common type of dementia is major NCD, an irreversible form of dementia caused by nerve cell deterioration.
- Providing a safe environment is a priority in the care of clients with major NCD.

Medications
- **Donepezil** (Aricept)
- **Galantamine** (galantamine hydrobromide; Reminyl [Canada]; Razadyne)
- **Memantine** (Ebixia [Canada]; Namenda)
- **Rivastigmine** (Exelon)
- **Tacrine** (Cognex)

Appendix A
Normal Laboratory Values

Test	Adult	Child	Infant/Newborn	Elder	Nursing Implications
Hematological					
Hgb (hemoglobin): mmol/L gm/dL	Male: 140-180 (14-18) Female: 120-160 (12-16) Pregnant: >110 (>11)	1-6 yr: 95-140 (9.5-14) 6-18 yr: 100-150 (10-15.5)	Neonate (0-28 days): 140-240 (14-24) Newborn 1-2 mo: 120-200 (12-20) 2-6 mo: 100-170 (10-17) 6 mo-1 yr: 95-140 (9.5-14)	Values slightly decreased	High-altitude living increases values. Drug therapy can alter values. Slight Hgb decreases normally occur during pregnancy.
Hct (hematocrit): volume fraction (%)	Male: 0.42-0.52 volume fraction (42-52) Female: 0.37-0.47 volume fraction (37-47) Pregnant: >0.33 volume fraction (>33)	6-12 yr: Male 0.31-0.38 (31-38); Female 0.32-0.39 (32-39) 12-18 yr: Male 0.31-0.41 (31-41); Female 0.32-0.39 (32-39)	Newborn: Male 0.37-0.47 (37-47); Female 0.38-0.48 (38-48) 15-30 days: Male 0.41-0.43 (41-43); Female 0.34-0.42 (34-42) 61-180 days: Male 0.31-0.38 (31-38); Female 0.31-0.39 (31-39) 6 mo-2 yr: Male 0.31-0.36 (31-36); Female 0.31-0.36 (31-36)	Values slightly decreased	Prolonged stasis from vasoconstriction secondary to the tourniquet can alter values. Abnormalities in RBC size may alter Hct values.
RBC (red blood cell) count: 10^{12}/L	Male: 4.7-6.1; Female: 4.2-5.4	1-6 yr: 4-5.5 6-18 yr: 4.5-5	Newborn: 4.8-7.1 2-8 wk: 4-6 2-6 mo: 3.5-5.5 6 mo-1 yr: 3.5-5.2	Same as adult	Never draw a specimen from an arm with an infusing IV. Exercise and high altitudes can cause an increase in values. Values are usually lower during pregnancy. Drug therapy can alter values.
WBC (white blood cell) count: $\times 10^{9}$/L (mm³)	Both genders: 5-10 (5,000-10,000)	≤2 yr: 6.2-17 (6,200-17,000) ≥2 yr: 5-10 (5,000-10,000)	Newborn (0-6 weeks): 9-30 (9,000-30,000)	Same as adult	Anesthetics, stress, exercise, and convulsions can cause increased values. Drug therapy can decrease values. 24-48 hr post partum: a count as high as 25,000 is normal.

Test	Adult	Child	Infant/Newborn	Elder	Nursing Implications
Platelet count: $\times 10^9$/L (mm³)	Both genders: 150-400 (150,000-400,000)	150-400 (150,000-400,000)	Premature infant: 100-300 (100,000-300,000) Newborn: 150-300 (150,000-300,000) Infant: 200-475 (200,000-475,000)	Same as adult	Living at high altitudes, exercising strenuously, or taking oral contraceptives may increase values. Decreased values may be caused by hemorrhage, DIC, reduced production of platelets, infections, use of prosthetic heart valves, and drugs (e.g., acetaminophen, aspirin, chemotherapy, H_2 blockers, INH, Levaquin, streptomycin, sulfonamides, thiazide diuretics).

HESI Hint: The laboratory values that are most important to know for the NCLEX-RN exam are Hgb, Hct, WBCs, Na^+, K^+, BUN, blood glucose, ABGs (arterial blood gases), bilirubin for newborns, and therapeutic range for PT and PTT.

Test	Adult	Child	Infant/Newborn	Elder	Nursing Implications
SED rate, ESR (erythrocyte sedimentation rate): mm/hr	Male: up to 15 Female: up to 20 Pregnant (all trimesters): up to 10	Same as adult	Newborn: 0-2	Same as adult	Pregnancy (second and third trimester) can cause elevations in ESR.
PT (prothrombin time): sec	Both genders: 11-12.5 Pregnant: slight ↓	Same as adult	Same as adult	Same as adult	PT is used to help regulate warfarin (Coumadin) dosages. Therapeutic range: 1.5-2 times normal or control.
PTT (partial thromboplastin time): sec (see APTT, below)	Both genders: 60-70 Pregnant: slight ↓	Same as adult	Same as adult	Same as adult	PTT is used to help regulate heparin dosages. Therapeutic range: 1.5-2.5 times normal or control.
INR (international normalized ratio)	Both genders: 0.8-1.2	Same as adult	Same as adult	Same as adult	Ideal INR value must be individualized. Typical values for certain clients are: Clients with atrial fibrillation and deep vein thrombosis: between 2.0 and 3.0 Clients with mechanical heart valves: between 3.0 and 4.0.
APTT (activated partial thromboplastin time): sec	Both genders: 30-40	Same as adult	Same as adult	Same as adult	APTT is used to help partially regulate heparin dosages. Therapeutic range: 1.5-2.5 times normal or control.

Test	Adult	Child	Infant/Newborn	Elder	Nursing Implications
Blood Chemistry					
Alkaline phosphatase: U/L	Both genders: 35-120	1-3 yr: 185-383 4-6 yr: 191-450 7-9 yr: 218-499 10-11 yr: Male 174-624; Female 169-657 12-13 yr: Male 245-584; Female 141-499 14-15 yr: Male 169-618; Female 103-283 16-19 yr: Male 98-317; Female 82-169		Slightly higher than adult	Hemolysis of specimen can cause falsely elevated values.
Albumin: g/dL	Both genders: 35-50 (3.5-5) Pregnant: slight ↓	40-59 (4.5-9)	Premature infant: 30-42 (3-4.2) Newborn: 35-54 (3.5-5.4) Infant: 44-54 (4.4-5.4)	Same as adult	No special preparation is needed.
Bilirubin total: mg/dL	Total: 0.3-1 Indirect: 0.2-0.8 Direct: 0.1-0.3	Same as adult	Newborn: 1-12	Same as adult	Client is kept NPO, except for water, for 8-12 hr before testing. Prevent hemolysis of blood during venipuncture. Do not shake tube; this can cause inaccurate values. Protect blood sample from bright light.
Hematological					
Calcium: mmol/L (mg/dL)	Both genders: 2.25-2.75 (9-10.5)	2.2-2.7 (8.8-10.8)	<10 days: 1.9-2.60 (7.6-10.4) Cord: 2.25-2.88 (9-11.5) 10 days-2 yr: 2.3-2.65 (9-10.6)	Values tend to decrease.	No special preparation is needed. Use of thiazide diuretics can cause increased calcium values.
Chloride: mmol/L (mEq/L)	Both genders: 98-106	90-110	Newborn: 96-106 Premature infant: 95-110	Same as adult	Do not collect from an arm with an infusing IV solution.
Cholesterol: mmol/L (mg/dL)	Both genders: <5.0 (<200)	10-11 yr: Male 3.10-5.90 (120-228); Female 3.16-6.26 (122-242)	Infant (7-12 mo): Male 2.15-5.30 (83-205); Female 1.76-5.59 (68-216) Newborn (0-1 mo): Male 0.98-4.50 (38-174); Female 1.45-5.04 (56-195)	Same as adult	Do not collect from an arm with an infusing IV solution.
CPK (creatine phosphokinase): IU/L	Male: 55-170 Female: 30-135	Same as adult	Newborn: 65-580	Same as adult	Specimen must not be stored before running test.

Test	Adult	Child	Infant/Newborn	Elder	Nursing Implications
Creatinine: mcmol/L (mg/dL)	Male: 53-106 (0.6-1.2); Female: 44-97 (0.5-1.1)	Child/Adolescent (1-18 yr): 18-62 (0.2-0.7)	Newborn (0-1 week): 53-97 (0.6-1.1) Infant (7 days-12 mo): 18-35 (0.2-0.4)	Decrease in muscle mass may cause decreased values	NPO for 8 hr before testing is preferred but not required. BUN-to-creatinine ratio of 20:1 indicates adequate kidney functioning.
Glucose: mmol/L (mg/dL)	Both genders: 4-6 (36-108)	≤2 yr: 3.3-5.5 (60-100) >2 yr: <6.1 (70-110)	Cord: 2.5-5.3 (45-96) Premature infant: 1.1-3.3 (20-60) Neonate (0-28 days): 1.7-3.3 (30-60) Infant (1 mo-2 yr): 2.2-5.0 (40-90) Newborn/Infant: 16-24	Normal range increases after age 50	Client is kept NPO, except for water, for 8 hr before testing. Stress, infection, and caffeine can cause increased values.
HCO₃⁻: mmol/L (mEq/L)	Both genders: 21-28	21-28	Newborn 13-22 Infant: 20-28	Same as adult	None
Iron: mcmol/L (mcg/dL)	Male: 14-32 (80-180) Female: 11-29 (60-160)	Child 4-10 yr: Male: 2.7-22.9 (15-128); Female: 5.0-21.8 (28-122)	Newborn: Male: 12.9-36.3 (72-203); Female: 13.4-42.1 (75-235)	Same as adult	NPO for 8 hr before test is preferred but not required.
TIBC (total iron binding capacity): mcmol/L (mcg/dL)	Both genders: 45-82 (250-460)	Same as adult	Newborn: 16.8-41.5 (94-232)	Same as adult	None
LDH (lactic dehydrogenase): U/L	Both genders: 100-190	60-170	Newborn: 160-450 Infant: 100-250	Same as adult	Do not give IM injections for 8-12 hr before test. Hemolysis of blood causes a false-positive result.
Potassium: mmol/L (mEq/L)	Both genders: 3.5-5	3.4-4.7	Newborn: 3.9-5.9 Infant: 4.1-5.3	Same as adult	Hemolysis of specimen can result in falsely elevated values. Exercise of the forearm with tourniquet in place may cause an increased potassium level.
Protein total: g/L (g/dL)	Both genders: 64-83 (6.4-8.3)	62-80 (6.2-8)	Premature infant: 42-76 (4.2-7.6) Newborn: 46-74 (4.6-7.4) Infant: 60-67 (6-6.7)	Same as adult	NPO for 8 hr before test is preferred but not required.
AST/SGOT (aspartate aminotransferase): U/L	0-35 Female slightly lower than adult male	3-6 yr: 15-50 6-12 yr: 10-50 12-18 yr: 10-40	0-5 days: 35-140 <3 yr: 15-60	Slightly higher than adult	Hemolysis of specimen can result in falsely elevated values. Exercise may cause an increased value.
ALT/SGPT (alanine aminotransferase): U/mL	Both genders: 4-36	Similar to adult	Values may be 2× as high as adults	Slightly higher than adult	Hemolysis of specimen can result in falsely elevated values. Exercise may cause an increased value.
Sodium: mEq/L	Both genders: 136-145	136-145	Newborn: 134-144 Infant: 134-150	Same as adult	Do not collect from an arm with an infusing IV solution.

Test	Adult	Child	Infant/Newborn	Elder	Nursing Implications
Triglycerides: mmol/L (mg/dL)	Male: 0.45-1.81 (40-160) Female: 0.40-1.52 (35-135)	4-6 yr: Male 0.36-1.31 (32-116); Female 0.36-1.31 (32-116) 7-9 yr: Male 0.32-1.46 (28-129); Female 0.32-1.46 (28-129) 10-11 yr: Male 0.27-1.55 (24-137); Female 0.44-1.58 (39-140) 12-13 yr: Male 0.27-1.64 (24-145); Female 0.42-1.47 (37-130) 14-15 yr: Male 0.38-1.86 (34-165); Female 0.43-1.52 (38-135) 16-19 yr: Male 0.38-1.58 (34-140); Female 0.42-1.58 (37-140)	0-3 yr: Male 0.31-1.41 (27-125); Female 0.31-1.41 (27-125)	Same as adult	Client is kept NPO for 12 hr before test. No alcohol for 24 hr before test.
BUN (blood urea nitrogen): mmol/L (mg/dL)	Both genders: 36-7.1 (10-20)	1.8-6.4 (5-18)	Newborn: 0.7-4.6 (2-13) Cord: 7.5-14.3 (21-40) Infant: 1.8-6.0 (5-17)	Slightly higher	None

Arterial Blood Chemistry					
pH	Both genders: 7.35-7.45	Child >2 yr: Same as adult	Newborn: 7.32-7.49 2 mo-2 yr: 7.34-7.46	Same as adult	Specimen must be heparinized. Specimen must be iced for transport. All air bubbles must be expelled from sample. Direct pressure to puncture site must be maintained.
PCO_2: mm Hg	Both genders: 35-45	Same as adult	<2 yr: 26-41	Same as adult	Specimen must be heparinized. Specimen must be iced for transport. All air bubbles must be expelled from sample. Direct pressure to puncture site must be maintained.
PO_2: mm Hg	Both genders: 80-100	Same as adult	Newborn/Infant: 16-24	Same as adult	Specimen must be heparinized. Specimen must be iced for transport. All air bubbles must be expelled from sample. Direct pressure to puncture site must be maintained.

Test	Adult	Child	Infant/Newborn	Elder	Nursing Implications
HCO_3^-: mmol/L (mEq/L)	Both genders: 21-28	Same as adult	Newborn/Infant: 16-24	Same as adult	Specimen must be heparinized. Specimen must be iced for transport. All air bubbles must be expelled from sample. Direct pressure to puncture site must be maintained.
O_2 saturation: %	Both genders: 95-100	Same as adult	Newborn: 40-90	95	Specimen must be heparinized. Specimen must be iced for transport. All air bubbles must be expelled from sample. Direct pressure to puncture site must be maintained.

From Pagana, T. J., & Pagana, K. D. (2013). *Mosby's Canadian manual of diagnostic and laboratory tests* (1st ed.). Toronto: Mosby; Pagana, T. J., & Pagana, K. D. (2013). *Mosby's manual of diagnostic and laboratory tests* (11th ed.). St Louis: Mosby.

BUN, Blood urea nitrogen; *DIC,* disseminated intravascular coagulation; *DVT,* deep vein thrombosis; *IM,* intramuscular; *INH,* isoniazid; *NPO,* nothing by mouth; *PCO_2,* carbon dioxide partial pressure; *PO_2,* oxygen partial pressure; *HCO_3^-,* bicarbonate.

Appendix B
Comparison of Three Types of Hepatitis

Characteristics	Hepatitis A (Infectious Hepatitis)	Hepatitis B (Serum Hepatitis)	Hepatitis C
Source of Infection	■ Contaminated food ■ Contaminated water or shellfish	■ Contaminated blood products ■ Contaminated needles or surgical instruments ■ Mother to child at birth	■ Contaminated blood products ■ Contaminated needles, IV drug use ■ Dialysis
Route of Infection	■ Oral ■ Fecal ■ Parenteral ■ Person to person	■ Parenteral ■ Oral ■ Fecal ■ Direct contact ■ Breast milk ■ Sexual contact	■ Parenteral ■ Sexual contact
Incubation Period	15-50 days	14-180 days	14-180 days (average)
Onset	Abrupt	Insidious	Insidious
Seasonal Variation	■ Autumn ■ Winter	All year	All year
Age Group Affected	■ Children ■ Young adults	Any age	Any age
Vaccine	Yes	Yes	No
Inoculation	Yes	Yes	Yes
Potential for Chronic Liver Disease	No	Yes	Yes
Immunity	Yes	Yes	No
Treatment	■ Prevention—hepatitis A (HAV) vaccine ■ Proper hand washing ■ Avoid contaminated food or water. ■ Obtain immunoglobulin within 14 days if exposed to the virus.	■ Prevention—hepatitis B (HBV) vaccine for high-risk groups ■ Antiviral and immunomodulating drugs	■ Subcutaneous pegylated interferon alpha once a week and oral ribavirin (Copegus, Rebetol) daily
Complications	Very few	■ Chronic hepatitis ■ Cirrhosis ■ Hepatitis D ■ Liver cancer	■ Chronic hepatitis ■ Cirrhosis ■ Liver cancer

Appendix C
Compare and Contrast: Parkinson's Disease, Myasthenia Gravis, and Multiple Sclerosis

	Parkinson's	Myasthenia Gravis	Multiple Sclerosis
Definition	Chronic, progressive neurodegenerative disorder	Autoimmune disorder of neuromuscular junction with fluctuating weakness of some skeletal muscles	Chronic, progressive, degenerative disorder Demyelination of nerve fibers of the brain and spinal cord
Patient	Peak onset in 70s, men	Onset between 10 and 65, women more common	Young to middle age, female, temperate climates
Etiology	Unknown, but with genetic and environmental components	Antibodies attack acetylcholine receptors, which prevents stimulation of muscle contraction	Unknown, may be related to viral, immunologic, and genetic factors
Signs and Symptoms	Gradual, insidious; may be unilateral; tremor more pronounced at rest Rigidity, bradykinesia, stooped posture, drooling, masked face, shuffling gait, jerky movements	Fluctuating weakness of skeletal muscles, strength restored after period of rest Primarily muscles of the eyes, mouth, and respiratory system Highly variable disorder	Insidious, gradual onset. Remissions and exacerbations: limb weakness, diplopia, numbness, tingling, neuropathic pain Decreased bowel, bladder function, sexual dysfunction, short-term memory cognitive changes
Nursing Management	Maximize neurologic function Maintain independence in ADL Optimize psychosocial aspects Safety	Optimize endurance Manage fatigue Avoid complications Maintain quality of life Safety	Maintain independence in ADL Maximize neuromuscular function Manage disabling fatigue Optimize psychosocial adjustment to illness Reduce exacerbating factors Safety
Medications	Dopaminergics Anticholinergics Antihistamine Monoamine oxidase inhibitors (MAIOs) Catechol-*O*-methyltransferase (COMT) inhibitors	Anticholinesterase drugs Corticosteroids Immunosuppressants	Corticosteroids Immunomodulators Cholinergics, anticholinergics Muscle relaxants Acetylcholinesterase inhibitors

ADL, activities of daily living.

NCLEX-RN Examination Practice Questions

Management/Leadership

1. **Which activity should the nurse delegate to an unlicensed assistive personnel (UAP)?**
   A. Check to see whether a client with cirrhosis can hear any better after discontinuation of an IV antibiotic.
   B. Encourage additional PO (by mouth) fluids for an elderly client with pneumonia who has developed a fever.
   C. Report the ability of a client with myasthenia gravis to manage the supper tray independently.
   D. Record the number of liquid stools of a client who received lactulose for an elevated NH_3 level.

HESI Test Question Approach			
Positive?		**YES**	**NO**
Key Words			
Rephrase			
Rule Out Choices			
A	B	C	D

2. **The nurse is assigning tasks to the UAP. Which client situation requires the RN to intervene?**
   A. A client with active tuberculosis who is leaving the room without a mask
   B. A client with dehydration who is requesting something to drink
   C. A client with asthma who complains of being anxious and unable to concentrate
   D. A client with chronic obstructive pulmonary disorder who is leaving the unit to smoke, even though the next intravenous piggyback is due

HESI Test Question Approach			
Positive?		**YES**	**NO**
Key Words			
Rephrase			
Rule Out Choices			
A	B	C	D

3. **When entering a client's room, the nurse finds the client threatening to cut herself with an unscrewed light bulb. What is the priority intervention?**
   A. Call in an extra nurse or UAP for the next shift.
   B. Assign one of the current UAPs to sit with the client.
   C. Move the client to another room with a roommate.
   D. Administer an as-needed (PRN) dose of lorazepam as prescribed.

HESI Test Question Approach			
Positive?		**YES**	**NO**
Key Words			
Rephrase			
Rule Out Choices			
A	B	C	D

4. A UAP is assisting with the care of eight clients on a postpartum unit. Which assignment should the nurse delegate to the UAP?
   A. Check fundal firmness and lochia for the clients who delivered vaginally.
   B. Take vital signs every 15 minutes for a client with preeclampsia.
   C. Provide breastfeeding instructions for a primigravida.
   D. Assist with daily care activities for the clients on bed rest.

HESI Test Question Approach			
Positive?		YES	NO
Key Words			
Rephrase			
Rule Out Choices			
A	B	C	D

Advanced Clinical Concepts

5. Which client is at the highest risk for respiratory complications?
   A. A 21-year-old client with dehydration and cerebral palsy who is dependent in daily activities
   B. A 60-year-old client who has had type 2 diabetes for 20 years and was admitted with cellulitis
   C. An obese 30-year-old client with hypertension who is noncompliant with the medication regimen
   D. A 40-year-old client who takes a loop diuretic, has a serum K^+ of 3.4 mmol/L (mEq/L), and complains of fatigue

HESI Test Question Approach			
Positive?		YES	NO
Key Words			
Rephrase			
Rule Out Choices			
A	B	C	D

6. A nurse working at a clinic finds a client in one of the examination rooms slumped over and apneic. The nurse notes an empty syringe and needle still in the client's arm. Which action has the highest priority?
   A. Call 911.
   B. Remove the syringe and needle.
   C. Assess for a pulse.
   D. Obtain the automated external defibrillator (AED).

HESI Test Question Approach			
Positive?		YES	NO
Key Words			
Rephrase			
Rule Out Choices			
A	B	C	D

7. A client who is immediately postoperative for aortic aneurysm repair has been receiving normal saline intravenously at 125 mL/hr. The nurse observes dark yellow urine. The hourly output for the past 3 hours was 50 mL, 32 mL, and 28 mL. What action should the nurse take?
   A. Administer a bolus D_5 ½ normal saline at 200 mL/hr.
   B. Contact the healthcare provider.
   C. Monitor output for another 2 hours.
   D. Draw blood samples for blood urea nitrogen (BUN) and creatinine labs.

HESI Test Question Approach

Positive?		YES	NO
Key Words			
Rephrase			
Rule Out Choices			
A	B	C	D

8. The RN is evaluating the effects of administration of fresh frozen plasma (FFP) on a client diagnosed with cirrhosis. Which finding(s) would indicate a positive outcome? (Select all that apply.)
   A. Blood urea nitrogen (BUN) 3.9 mmol/L (11 mg/dL); creatinine 62 mcmol/L (0.7 mg/dL)
   B. Hemoglobin level of 100 mmol/L (10 gm/dL)
   C. Return of temperature to normal
   D. Decreased bleeding from the gums
   E. Negative guaiac for occult bleeding

HESI Test Question Approach

Positive?			YES	NO
Key Words				
Rephrase				
Rule Out Choices				
A	B	C	D	E

9. A client's arterial blood gas results are as follows: pH 7.29, P_{CO_2} 55 mm Hg, and H_{CO_3} 26 mEq/L. Which compensatory response should the nurse expect to see?
   A. Respiratory rate of 30 breaths/min
   B. Apical rate of 120 beats/min
   C. Potassium level of 5.8 mmol/L (mEq/L)
   D. Complaints of pounding headache

HESI Test Question Approach

Positive?		YES	NO
Key Words			
Rephrase			
Rule Out Choices			
A	B	C	D

10. **A client with chronic back pain is not receiving adequate pain relief from oral analgesics. Which alternative action should the nurse explore to promote the client's independence?**
    A. Ask the healthcare provider to increase the analgesic dosage.
    B. Obtain a prescription for a second analgesic, to be given by the IV route.
    C. Consider the client's receptivity to complementary therapy.
    D. Encourage counseling to prevent future addiction.

HESI Test Question Approach			
Positive?		YES	NO
Key Words			
Rephrase			
Rule Out Choices			
A	B	C	D

Maternal/Newborn Nursing

11. **A client at 41 weeks' gestation who is in active labor calls the nurse to report that her membranes have ruptured. The nurse performs a vaginal examination and discovers that the umbilical cord has prolapsed. Which intervention should the nurse implement first?**
    A. Elevate the presenting fetal part off the cord.
    B. Cover the cord with sterile moist NS gauze.
    C. Prepare for an emergency cesarean delivery.
    D. Administer O_2 by facemask at 10 L/min.

HESI Test Question Approach			
Positive?		YES	NO
Key Words			
Rephrase			
Rule Out Choices			
A	B	C	D

12. **A client at 39 weeks' gestation plans to have an epidural block when labor is established. What intervention(s) should the nurse implement to prevent side effects? (Select all that apply.)**
    A. Teach about the procedure and effects of the epidural.
    B. Place the client in a chair next to the bed.
    C. Administer a bolus of 500 mL of normal saline solution.
    D. Monitor the fetal heart rate and contractions continuously.
    E. Assist the client to empty her bladder every 2 hours.

HESI Test Question Approach				
Positive?			YES	NO
Key Words				
Rephrase				
Rule Out Choices				
A	B	C	D	E

13. A female client presents in the emergency department with right lower quadrant abdominal pain and pain in her right shoulder. She has no vaginal bleeding, and her last menses was 6 weeks ago. Which actions should the nurse take first?
   A. Assess for abdominal rebound pain, distention, and fever.
   B. Obtain vital signs and IV access, and notify the healthcare provider.
   C. Observe for recent musculoskeletal injury, bruising, or abuse.
   D. Collect specimens for pregnancy test, hemoglobin, and white blood cell count.

HESI Test Question Approach

Positive?			YES	NO
Key Words				
Rephrase				
Rule Out Choices				
A	B		C	D

14. A nurse has been assigned a pregnant client who has heart disease. The client's condition has been diagnosed as New York Heart Association (NYHA) Class II cardiac disease. What important fact(s) about activities of daily living while pregnant should the nurse teach this client? (Select all that apply.)
   A. Increase fiber in the diet.
   B. Avoid sexual intercourse.
   C. Notify the healthcare provider if her rings do not fit.
   D. Maintain bed rest with bathroom privileges.
   E. Start a low-impact aerobic program.

HESI Test Question Approach

Positive?				YES	NO
Key Words					
Rephrase					
Rule Out Choices					
A	B	C	D	E	

Medical-Surgical: Renal

15. A client is returning to the unit after an intravenous pyelogram (IVP). Which intervention should the nurse include in the client's plan of care?
   A. Maintain bed rest.
   B. Increase fluid intake.
   C. Monitor for hematuria.
   D. Continue NPO (nothing by mouth) status.

HESI Test Question Approach

Positive?			YES	NO
Key Words				
Rephrase				
Rule Out Choices				
A	B		C	D

16. The nurse is teaching a client who has chronic urinary tract infections about a prescription for ciprofloxacin (Cipro) 500 mg PO bid (twice daily). What side effect(s) could the client expect while taking this medication? (Select all that apply.)
   A. Photosensitivity
   B. Dyspepsia
   C. Diarrhea
   D. Urinary frequency
   E. Pernicious anemia

HESI Test Question Approach			
Positive?		YES	NO
Key Words			
Rephrase			
Rule Out Choices			
A	B	C	D	E

17. Which client complaint of pain requires the nurse's immediate intervention?
   A. Bladder pain while receiving a continuous saline irrigant 2 hours after a transurethral prostatic resection
   B. Incisional pain on postoperative day 3 after a nephrectomy; the client requests an as-needed (PRN) oral pain medication
   C. Flank pain that is partially relieved when the client passes a renal calculus
   D. Bladder spasms after draining 1,000 mL of urine during insertion of an indwelling catheter

HESI Test Question Approach			
Positive?		YES	NO
Key Words			
Rephrase			
Rule Out Choices			
A	B	C	D

18. A male client with a peritoneal dialysis catheter calls to report that he feels poorly and has a fever. What is the best response by the clinic nurse?
   A. Encourage him to come to the clinic today for assessment.
   B. Instruct him to increase his fluid intake to 3 L/day.
   C. Review his medication regimen for compliance.
   D. Inquire about his recent dietary intake of protein and iron.

HESI Test Question Approach			
Positive?		YES	NO
Key Words			
Rephrase			
Rule Out Choices			
A	B	C	D

19. The nurse is reviewing the cardiac markers for a client who was admitted immediately after reporting chest pain. Which marker is the best to determine cardiac damage?

A. Troponin levels
B. Myoglobin level
C. Creatine kinase-MB level
D. Lactate dehydrogenase (LDH) level

HESI Test Question Approach			
Positive?		**YES**	**NO**
Key Words			
Rephrase			
Rule Out Choices			
A	**B**	**C**	**D**

20. The nurse is providing discharge instructions to a client who has been diagnosed with angina pectoris. Which instruction is most important?

A. Avoid activity that involves the Valsalva maneuver.
B. Seek emergency treatment if chest pain persists after the third nitroglycerin dose.
C. Rest for 30 minutes after having chest pain before resuming activity.
D. Keep extra nitroglycerin in an airtight, light-resistant bottle.

HESI Test Question Approach			
Positive?		**YES**	**NO**
Key Words			
Rephrase			
Rule Out Choices			
A	**B**	**C**	**D**

21. The nurse is providing discharge teaching for a client who has been prescribed diltiazem. Which dietary instruction has the highest priority?

A. Maintain a low-sodium diet.
B. Eat a banana each morning.
C. Ingest high-fiber foods daily.
D. Avoid grapefruit products.

HESI Test Question Approach			
Positive?		**YES**	**NO**
Key Words			
Rephrase			
Rule Out Choices			
A	**B**	**C**	**D**

22. **The nurse is teaching a young adult female who has a history of Raynaud's disease how to control her pain. What information should the nurse offer?**
    A. Take oral analgesics at regularly spaced intervals.
    B. Avoid extremes of heat and cold.
    C. Limit foods and fluids that contain caffeine.
    D. Keep the affected extremities in a dependent position.

HESI Test Question Approach			
Positive?		YES	NO
Key Words			
Rephrase			
Rule Out Choices			
A	B	C	D

23. **The clinic nurse is caring for a client taking warfarin for atrial fibrillation. Which client need should the nurse give highest priority?**
    A. Having protamine sulfate available
    B. Teaching the client the importance of walking 10,000 steps daily
    C. Encouraging the client to eat Brussels sprouts and cabbage
    D. Monitoring the platelet count for indications of thrombocytopenia

HESI Test Question Approach			
Positive?		YES	NO
Key Words			
Rephrase			
Rule Out Choices			
A	B	C	D

Medical-Surgical: Respiratory

24. **A client who was admitted to the hospital with cancer of the larynx is scheduled for a laryngectomy tomorrow. What is the client's priority learning need tonight?**
    A. Anticipated body image changes
    B. Pain management expectations
    C. Communication techniques
    D. Postoperative nutritional needs

HESI Test Question Approach			
Positive?		YES	NO
Key Words			
Rephrase			
Rule Out Choices			
A	B	C	D

25. A victim of a motor vehicle collision is dead on arrival at the emergency department. What action should the nurse take to assist the spouse with this crisis?
   A. Ask whether there is family, friends, or clergy to call.
   B. Talk about the former relationship with the spouse.
   C. Provide education about the stages of grief and loss.
   D. Assess the spouse's level of anxiety.

HESI Test Question Approach

Positive?		YES	NO
Key Words			
Rephrase			
Rule Out Choices			
A	B	C	D

26. The nurse is planning to lead a seminar for community health nurses on violence against women during pregnancy. Which statement describes an appropriate technique for assessing for violence?
   A. Women should be assessed only if they are part of a high-risk group.
   B. Women may be assessed in the presence of young children but not intimate partners.
   C. Women should be assessed once during pregnancy.
   D. Women should be reassessed face to face by a nurse as the pregnancy progresses.

HESI Test Question Approach

Positive?		YES	NO
Key Words			
Rephrase			
Rule Out Choices			
A	B	C	D

27. The charge nurse reminds clients on the mental health unit that breakfast is at 8 AM, medications are given at 9 AM, and group therapy sessions begin at 10 AM. Which treatment modality has been implemented?
   A. Milieu therapy
   B. Behavior modification
   C. Peer therapy
   D. Problem solving

HESI Test Question Approach

Positive?		YES	NO
Key Words			
Rephrase			
Rule Out Choices			
A	B	C	D

28. The nurse is accompanying a client to the radiography department when he becomes panic stricken at the elevator and states, "I can't get on that elevator." Which action should the nurse take first?
    A. Ask one more staff member to ride in the elevator.
    B. Offer a prescribed antianxiety medication.
    C. Begin desensitization about riding the elevator.
    D. Affirm the client's fears about riding the elevator.

HESI Test Question Approach

Positive?		YES	NO
Key Words			

Rephrase

Rule Out Choices

A	B	C	D

29. A client who experiences frequent nightmares and somnambulism is found one night trying to strangle his roommate. Which intervention is the nurse's highest priority?
    A. Give the client a sedative or hypnotic.
    B. Administer an antipsychotic.
    C. Assign a UAP to sit with the client.
    D. Process with both clients about event.

HESI Test Question Approach

Positive?		YES	NO
Key Words			

Rephrase

Rule Out Choices

A	B	C	D

30. The nurse is updating the plan of care for a client who has a borderline personality disorder. Which intervention is most important to implement?
    A. Always assign the same nurse to care for the client.
    B. Avoid challenging inappropriate behavior.
    C. Limit the client's contact with other clients.
    D. Remove consequences for acting-out behaviors.

HESI Test Question Approach

Positive?		YES	NO
Key Words			

Rephrase

Rule Out Choices

A	B	C	D

31. A female adolescent is admitted to the mental health unit for anorexia nervosa. In planning care, what is the nurse's highest priority?
    A. Teach the client the importance of self-expression.
    B. Supervise the client's activities closely.
    C. Include the client in daily group therapy.
    D. Facilitate social interactions with others.

HESI Test Question Approach

Positive?		YES	NO
Key Words			
Rephrase			
Rule Out Choices			
A	B	C	D

32. The charge nurse is planning the daily schedule for clients on the mental health unit. A male client who is manic should be assigned to which activity?
    A. A basketball game in the gym
    B. Jogging at least 1 mile daily
    C. A table tennis game with a peer
    D. Group activity with the art therapist

HESI Test Question Approach

Positive?		YES	NO
Key Words			
Rephrase			
Rule Out Choices			
A	B	C	D

Leadership and Delegation

33. A nurse is planning the client assignments for the night shift. The nursing team includes a registered nurse, a licensed practical nurse, and two unlicensed assistive personnel (UAP). Which duty (or duties) could be delegated to the UAPs? (Select all that apply.)
    A. Transport a client who has had a stroke to the radiology department for a computed tomography (CT) scan.
    B. Retrieve a unit of packed cells from the blood bank for a transfusion.
    C. Bathe a 25-year-old client with sickle cell disease who has multiple IV lines and a patient-controlled analgesia pump.
    D. Turn a 92-year-old client who has end-stage heart failure and a do-not-resuscitate order.
    E. Contact the healthcare provider for a client with a fingerstick blood glucose level of 2.72 mmol/L (49 mg/dL).

HESI Test Question Approach

Positive?			YES	NO
Key Words				
Rephrase				
Rule Out Choices				
A	B	C	D	E

34. A hospitalized client has been newly diagnosed with type 2 diabetes. Which task(s) can the RN delegate to the UAP? (Select all that apply.)
A. Contacting the dietitian for a prescribed consult
B. Reporting the client's insulin injection technique
C. Obtaining the fingerstick blood glucose level before each meal and at bedtime
D. Reminding the client to dry the toes carefully after a shower
E. Talking to the client about foods that raise the blood glucose level

HESI Test Question Approach				
Positive?			YES	NO
Key Words				
Rephrase				
Rule Out Choices				
A	B	C	D	E

35. The home health nurse evaluates the insulin preparation and administration technique of a 36-year-old male client newly diagnosed with diabetes. The client has been prescribed insulin: lispro (Humalog) pen 10 units subcutaneously ac and Lantus 45 units subcutaneously once daily in AM. Which finding indicates that the client needs further education?
A. He mixes Lantus and lispro in the same syringe for the AM dose.
B. He leaves the insulin syringe in place for 5 seconds after injection.
C. He stores the opened insulin vials at room temperature in the cabinet.
D. He recaps and disposes of the single-use insulin syringe.

HESI Test Question Approach			
Positive?		YES	NO
Key Words			
Rephrase			
Rule Out Choices			
A	B	C	D

36. At change of shift, the charge nurse assigns the UAP four clients. The RN should direct the UAP to take vitals sign on which client first?
A. The 89-year-old with chronic obstructive pulmonary disease who is resting quietly on 2 L of oxygen and who needs assistance with a bath
B. The client who returned from endoscopy about 30 minutes ago and is requesting something to eat
C. The client newly diagnosed with type 2 diabetes who had a fingerstick glucose level of 4.2 mmol/L (75 mg/dL) and needs help with breakfast
D. The newly admitted client with rheumatoid arthritis who needs hand splints reapplied to both hands

HESI Test Question Approach			
Positive?		YES	NO
Key Words			
Rephrase			
Rule Out Choices			
A	B	C	D

37. After change-of-shift report, the nurse reviews her assignments. Which client should the nurse assess first?

A. The elderly client receiving palliative care for heart failure who complains of constipation and nervousness

B. The adult client admitted for possible pneumonia with a heart rate of 110 and a respiratory rate of 24

C. The middle-aged client with end-stage renal failure whose urinary output has been 95 mL for the past 8 hours

D. The client who is 2 days postoperative from a thoracotomy and who has chest tubes, is on oxygen at 3 L/min, and has a respiratory rate of 12 breaths/min

HESI Test Question Approach			
Positive?		YES	NO
Key Words			
Rephrase			
Rule Out Choices			
A	B	C	D

38. The nurse is reviewing the laboratory values of her assigned clients. Which client has an abnormal laboratory report that the nurse should immediately call to the healthcare provider?

A. The client who is post splenectomy after a motor vehicle accident and has a hemoglobin of 109 mmol/L (10.9 g/dL)

B. The client receiving warfarin (Coumadin) who has an international normalized ratio (INR) of 2.3

C. The 38-year-old client who is 24 hours post thyroidectomy and has a total calcium level of 2.35 mmol/L (9.4 mg/dL)

D. The newly admitted client with a blood urea nitrogen (BUN) of 10.7 mmol/L (30 mg/dL) and a creatinine of 97 mcmol/L (1.1 mg/dL)

HESI Test Question Approach			
Positive?		YES	NO
Key Words			
Rephrase			
Rule Out Choices			
A	B	C	D

39. The nurse receives change-of-shift report on her four acute care clients. Which action should the nurse take first?

A. Contact the healthcare provider for a prescription for an antiemetic on a postoperative client who has been vomiting.

B. Notify a family member of a client's impending transfer to the intensive care unit for angina and ST segment changes.

C. Inform the healthcare provider of a potassium level of 5.2 mmol/L (mEq/L) in the client with end-stage renal disease.

D. Begin assessment rounds, starting with the palliative care client having a diagnosis of congestive failure

HESI Test Question Approach			
Positive?		YES	NO
Key Words			
Rephrase			
Rule Out Choices			
A	B	C	D

40. **The emergency department staff nurse is assigned four clients. Which client should the nurse assess first?**
    A. A preschooler with a barking cough, an O_2 saturation of 93% on room air, and occasional inspiratory stridor
    B. A 10-month-old infant with a tympanic temperature of 38.9 °C (102 °F) and green nasal drainage who is pulling at her ears
    C. A crying 8-month-old with a harsh, paroxysmal cough; an audible expiratory wheeze; and mild retractions
    D. A clingy 3-year-old who has a sore throat and drooling and whose tongue is slightly protruding from his mouth

HESI Test Question Approach			
Positive?		YES	NO
Key Words			
Rephrase			
Rule Out Choices			
A	B	C	D

41. **The outpatient clinic nurse is reviewing phone messages from last night. Which client should the nurse call back first?**
    A. A woman at 30 weeks' gestation who has been diagnosed with mild pre-eclampsia; she was unable to relieve her heartburn
    B. A woman at 24 weeks' gestation who was crying about painful vulvar lesions and urinary frequency for the past 8 hours
    C. A woman at 12 weeks' gestation who was recently discharged from the hospital with hyperemesis gravidarum; she had had two episodes of vomiting in 6 hours
    D. A woman with type 1 diabetes who tested positive with a home pregnancy kit; she was worried about managing her diabetes

HESI Test Question Approach			
Positive?		YES	NO
Key Words			
Rephrase			
Rule Out Choices			
A	B	C	D

42. **The clinic nurse suspects that a 2-year-old child is being abused. Which assessment finding(s) would support this? (Select all that apply.)**
    A. Petechiae in a straight line on the chest
    B. Gray-blue pigmented areas on the sacral region
    C. Bald patches on the scalp
    D. Ear tugging and crying
    E. Symmetrical burns on the hands

HESI Test Question Approach				
Positive?			YES	NO
Key Words				
Rephrase				
Rule Out Choices				
A	B	C	D	E

43. The nurse is caring for a client who had a thoracotomy 48 hours earlier and now has left lower lobe chest tubes. The nurse notes that a chest tube is not tidaling. Which action should the nurse take first?

A. Check for kinks in the chest drainage system.
B. Assess the heart rate and blood pressure.
C. Notify the rapid response team immediately.
D. Momentarily disconnect from wall suction.

HESI Test Question Approach			
Positive?		**YES**	**NO**
Key Words			
Rephrase			
Rule Out Choices			
A	**B**	**C**	**D**

44. While the nurse is caring for a client who has had a myocardial infarction, the monitor alarm sounds, and the nurse notes ventricular fibrillation. What should be the nurse's first course of action?

A. Notify the healthcare provider.
B. Increase the oxygen concentration.
C. Assess the client's level of consciousness.
D. Prepare to defibrillate the client.

HESI Test Question Approach			
Positive?		**YES**	**NO**
Key Words			
Rephrase			
Rule Out Choices			
A	**B**	**C**	**D**

45. The healthcare provider has prescribed the removal of a client's internal jugular central line catheter. To remove the catheter safely, the nurse should give which intervention(s) the highest priority? (Select all that apply.)

A. Carefully remove the Bioderm dressing.
B. Place the client in the Trendelenburg position.
C. Send the catheter tip to the laboratory for a culture and sensitivity.
D. Have the client take a deep breath during removal.
E. Apply pressure for 20 minutes after removal of the catheter.

HESI Test Question Approach				
Positive?			**YES**	**NO**
Key Words				
Rephrase				
Rule Out Choices				
A	**B**	**C**	**D**	**E**

46. The nurse who usually works on the orthopedic surgery unit is floating to a cardiovascular unit. Which client would be best to assign to the float nurse?
    A. Client scheduled for a heart catheterization this morning
    B. Client admitted last night for chest pain.
    C. Client who is 1 day postoperative for popliteal bypass surgery
    D. Client with heart failure and scheduled for a stress test today.

HESI Test Question Approach		
Positive?	YES	NO
Key Words		
Rephrase		
Rule Out Choices		
A	B	C	D

47. The nurse is admitting a client who is a paraplegic and has a nonhealing pressure ulcer with a possible methicillin-resistant *Staphylococcus aureus* infection. A PN and UAP are assigned to the nurse's team. Which tasks should be delegated to the PN? (Select all that apply.)
    A. Place the client in isolation.
    B. Complete a dressing change.
    C. Assess and document the wound.
    D. Insert a urinary catheter.
    E. Administer oral pain medications.

HESI Test Question Approach		
Positive?	YES	NO
Key Words		
Rephrase		
Rule Out Choices		
A	B	C	D	E

48. The nursing supervisor calls the charge nurse on a step-down unit about the need to open up a bed for a transfer of an unstable patient from the medical unit. Which client should the nurse transfer to the medical unit to receive this unstable client?
    A. A client admitted for an ST-elevation myocardial infarction (STEMI) who just returned from having a cardiac catheterization performed
    B. A client diagnosed with congestive heart failure who is receiving furosemide IV twice a day
    C. A client with possible Guillain-Barré syndrome who may need an exchange transfusion
    D. A client in hypertensive crisis who is prescribed a sodium nitroprusside drip

HESI Test Question Approach		
Positive?	YES	NO
Key Words		
Rephrase		
Rule Out Choices		
A	B	C	D

49. When accessing the Pyxis, the nurse finds chlorpropamide in the drawer instead of the expected chlorpromazine. Which actions should the nurse take? (Select all that apply.)
  A. Remove the tablets of chlorpropamide.
  B. Notify the pharmacy about the mistake.
  C. Place an incident occurrence report.
  D. Be extra vigilant because pharmacy is making mistakes.
  E. Place a warning note on the Pyxis machine.

HESI Test Question Approach			
Positive?		YES	NO
Key Words			
Rephrase			
Rule Out Choices			
A	B	C	D	E

50. The nurse is calling the healthcare provider (HCP) about a client's current needs. What is the best way to communicate?
  A. Call the HCP with the request and a recommendation.
  B. Use the SBAR (situation, background, assessment, recommendation) tool for communication.
  C. Send a text message or page with the needed order.
  D. Ask the HCP to come back to the unit to discuss the client's needs.

HESI Test Question Approach			
Positive?		YES	NO
Key Words			
Rephrase			
Rule Out Choices			
A	B	C	D

51. The healthcare provider plans to do a paracentesis on a client with cirrhosis in 1 hour. In what order should the nurse perform the following activities?
  A. Ensure that the informed consent has been obtained.
  B. Measure the client's abdominal girth.
  C. Have the client empty his or her bladder.
  D. Assemble needed equipment.
  E. Administer oral pain medication.

HESI Test Question Approach			
Positive?		YES	NO
Key Words			
Rephrase			
Rule Out Choices			
A	B	C	D	E

52. **The nurse receives report on a client from the emergency department with a diagnosis of pneumonia. Which intervention has the highest priority?**
    A. Obtain blood cultures.
    B. Initiate prescribed antibiotics.
    C. Place the client in isolation.
    D. Obtain an accurate weight.

HESI Test Question Approach			
Positive?		YES	NO
Key Words			
Rephrase			
Rule Out Choices			
A	B	C	D

53. **The nurse is part of the triage team at a disaster. Which client should be seen first?**
    A. A 90-year-old woman with a crushed pelvis and head injuries
    B. A 21-year-old man screaming in pain from a broken leg
    C. A 30-year-old woman with a flail chest secondary to a puncture wound
    D. A 12-year-old crying with multiple small lacerations

HESI Test Question Approach			
Positive?		YES	NO
Key Words			
Rephrase			
Rule Out Choices			
A	B	C	D

54. **The triage nurse in the emergency room is assessing four (4) clients. Which client requires the most immediate intervention?**
    A. The adult client who arrived via ambulance with numbness and tingling of his left arm and face
    B. The adult client who had a seizure at home who is sleeping on his left side..
    C. The 60-year-old client who complains of frequent urination and has a blood sugar of 16.7 mmol/L (300 mg/dL)
    D. The middle-aged client who presents with severe unilateral back pain and previous history of kidney stones

HESI Test Question Approach			
Positive?		YES	NO
Key Words			
Rephrase			
Rule Out Choices			
A	B	C	D

55. After a change-of-shift report on an orthopedic floor, which client should the nurse assess first?
   A. A client who had surgery yesterday and has a temperature of 37.6 °C (99.7 °F)
   B. A client who is complaining of numbness and tingling distal to the fracture site
   C. A client who had a left leg amputation and states he is experiencing pain in the left foot
   D. A client who is extremely upset with the care and is requesting to speak to the manager

HESI Test Question Approach

Positive?		YES	NO
Key Words			
Rephrase			
Rule Out Choices			
A	B	C	D

56. The nurse is administering medications to a client admitted for an overdose and a history of substance abuse. Which intervention(s) are a priority to include in this client's plan of care? (Select all that apply.)
   A. Allow the client to take medications independently.
   B. Ensure that all medications have been swallowed before leaving the client's room.
   C. Request that oral pain medications be changed from tablet to oral suspension.
   D. Administer Romazicon as prescribed every 6 hours around the clock.
   E. Administer all medications to the client via the intravenous route.

HESI Test Question Approach

Positive?			YES	NO
Key Words				
Rephrase				
Rule Out Choices				
A	B	C	D	E

57. The nurse is returning phone calls to clients who are cared for at an outpatient mental health center. Which client should the nurse call first?
   A. The young mother diagnosed with schizophrenia who is hearing voices saying that they are pursuing her children
   B. The elderly man at an assisted living facility who says he wants to end it all
   C. The female client diagnosed with bipolar disorder who has not slept for 48 hours.
   D. The teenager diagnosed with bulimia whose mother called and reported that she found her daughter purging

HESI Test Question Approach

Positive?		YES	NO
Key Words			
Rephrase			
Rule Out Choices			
A	B	C	D

58. An 18-year-old woman is being discharged after delivering a healthy baby. She has a cousin whose baby died from sudden infant death syndrome (SIDS). The client seems to know many of the precautions to take. Which information does the nurse need to correct?
    A. Always place infants on their backs to sleep.
    B. Room sharing has been shown to decrease SIDS.
    C. Keep the crib free of stuffed animals and crib pads.
    D. Sleeping with the baby can alert the mother to changes.

HESI Test Question Approach			
Positive?		YES	NO
Key Words			
Rephrase			
Rule Out Choices			
A	B	C	D

59. A 4-year-old admitted with pneumonia weighs 18 kg. The healthcare provider has prescribed vancomycin 40 mg/kg/day IV. The order states to divide the dose and give it three times daily. How many milligrams of vancomycin should the child receive in each dose? (Round the answer to the nearest whole number.)

    _____ mg/dose

60. The nurse needs to initiate an IV on an 8-year-old child. Which intervention is appropriate?
    A. Start the IV in the treatment room, not the child's room.
    B. Apply a lidocaine-based cream for a few minutes before starting the IV.
    C. Ask the parents to leave the room while performing the procedure.
    D. Encourage the child to use guided imagery to cope.

HESI Test Question Approach			
Positive?		YES	NO
Key Words			
Rephrase			
Rule Out Choices			
A	B	C	D

Answers and Rationales

(Correct answers are underlined.)

Management/Leadership

1. **Which activity should the nurse delegate to an unlicensed assistive personnel (UAP)?**

Rationales:
A. *Check to see whether a client with cirrhosis can hear any better today after discontinuation of an IV antibiotic.*
This requires assessment about ototoxicity, which is beyond the scope of practice of a UAP.
B. *Encourage additional PO (by mouth) fluids for an elderly client with pneumonia who has developed a fever.*
These directions are not sufficiently clear and detailed for the UAP to perform the task.
C. *Report the ability of a client with myasthenia gravis to manage the supper tray independently.*
This requires assessment of the client's clinical status, which is beyond the scope of the UAP.
D. <u>*Record the number of liquid stools of a client who has received lactulose for an increased NH_3 level.*</u>
This task encompasses basic care, elimination, and intake and output; it does not require judgment or the expertise of the nurse and can be performed by the UAP.

2. **The nurse is assigning tasks to the UAP. Which client situation requires the RN to intervene?**

Rationales:
A. *A client with active TB who is leaving the room without a mask*
A UAP can be delegated to provide a box of masks or to direct the client back to the room.
B. *A client with dehydration who is requesting something to drink*
A UAP can be directed to provide specific types and amounts of fluids.
C. <u>*A client with asthma who complains of being anxious and unable to concentrate*</u>
This client requires assessment and is at risk for airway compromise, which also requires assessment, so the nurse should attend to this client.
D. *A client with chronic obstructive pulmonary disorder who is leaving the unit to smoke, even though the next IVPB is due*
A UAP can ask the client to delay leaving the unit.

3. **When entering a client's room, the nurse finds the client threatening to cut herself with an unscrewed light bulb. What is the priority intervention?**

Rationales:
A. *Call in an extra nurse or UAP for the next shift.*
The charge nurse should plan ahead for staffing, but the immediate focus should be the client's safety now.
B. <u>*Assign one of the current UAPs to sit with the client.*</u>
Because the client is at risk for suicide, the charge nurse should assign a staff member to stay with the client.
C. *Move the client to another room with a roommate.*
This will not ensure the client's safety; also, a staff member, not another client, must be present with the client at all times.
D. *Administer an as-needed (PRN) dose of lorazepam as prescribed*
Although the client may be anxious, this is not a priority intervention that would ensure her safety.

4. **A UAP is assisting with the care of eight clients on a postpartum unit. Which assignment should the nurse delegate to the UAP?**

Rationales:
A. *Check fundal firmness and lochia for the clients who delivered vaginally.*
Assessment is a responsibility of the nurse.
B. *Take vital signs every 15 minutes for a client with preeclampsia.*
This is a high-risk patient who needs to be evaluated by a licensed nurse.
C. *Provide breastfeeding instructions for a primigravida.*
Teaching is the responsibility of the RN.
D. <u>*Assist with daily care activities for the clients on bed rest.*</u>
This is the most appropriate assignment for the UAP. The RN should delegate daily care activities to the UAP based on the RN's assessments of each client's needs.

Advanced Clinical Concepts

5. **Which client is at the highest risk for respiratory complications?**

Rationales:
A. <u>*A 21-year-old client with dehydration and cerebral palsy who is dependent in daily activities*</u>
A client with dehydration and cerebral palsy (characterized by uncoordinated, spastic muscle movements) that affects activities of daily living independence is at increased risk for respiratory problems because of impaired mobility and impaired swallowing.
B. *A 60-year-old client who has had type 2 diabetes for 20 years and was admitted with cellulitis*
This older client is more at risk for renal, cardiac, and vascular complications.
C. *An obese 30-year-old client with hypertension who is noncompliant with the medication regimen*
An obese adult who is noncompliant with antihypertensive medications is more at risk for cardiac or cerebral events than for respiratory problems.

D. **A 40-year-old client who takes a loop diuretic, has a serum K+ of 3.4 mmol/L (mEq/L), and complains of fatigue**
This middle-aged adult is hypokalemic and fatigued but is not at high risk for respiratory problems.

6. **A nurse working at a clinic finds a client in one of the examination rooms slumped over and apneic. The nurse notes an empty syringe and needle still in the client's arm. Which action has the highest priority?**

Rationales:
A. **Call 911.**
Calling for assistance is a high priority but not the highest.
B. **Remove the syringe and needle.**
The syringe and needle should be removed and possibly sent to a laboratory for analysis of the contents, but this is not a priority.
C. _Assess for a pulse._
Assessing for a pulse is the highest priority to determine whether cardiopulmonary resuscitation (CPR) needs to be initiated.
D. **Obtain the AED.**
This action is needed only if there is no pulse detected.

7. **A client who is immediately postoperative for abdominal aortic aneurysm repair has been receiving normal saline intravenously at 125 mL/hr. The nurse observes dark yellow urine. The hourly output for the past 3 hours was 50 mL, 32 mL, and 28 mL. What action should the nurse take?**

Rationales:
A. **Administer a bolus D5 ½ normal saline at 200 mL/hr.**
This action is not recommended because hypertonic solutions are prescribed for fluid and electrolyte imbalances and cause an osmotic movement of fluids into the vasculature.
B. _Contact the healthcare provider._
Low urinary output may be a serious problem and requires more immediate intervention from the healthcare provider.
C. **Monitor output for another 2 hours.**
Urine output has been monitored and may indicate dehydration, which can lead to more serious complications.
D. **Draw blood samples for blood urea nitrogen (BUN) and creatinine labs.**
The BUN and creatinine should be evaluated, but these tests are not the immediate priority.

8. **The RN is evaluating the effects of administration of fresh frozen plasma (FFP) on a client diagnosed with cirrhosis. Which finding(s) would indicate a positive outcome? (Select all that apply.)**

Rationales:
A. **Blood urea nitrogen (BUN) 3.9 mmol/L (11 mg/dL); creatinine 62 mcmol/L (0.7mg/dL)**
These values are not affected by administration of FFP.
B. **Hemoglobin level of 100 mmol/L (10 gm/dL)**
FFP does not affect hemoglobin levels.
C. **Return of temperature to normal**
Although monitoring the client's temperature is important, FFP does not have a direct effect on this parameter.
D. _Decreased bleeding from the gums_
FFP replaces clotting factors; therefore, detecting obvious bleeding provides valuable information.
E. _Negative guaiac for occult bleeding_
FFP replaces clotting factors: therefore, detecting occult (hidden) bleeding provides valuable information.

9. **A client's arterial blood gas results are as follows: pH 7.29, Pco$_2$ 55 mm Hg, and Hco$_3$ 26 mEq/L. Which compensatory response should the nurse expect to see?**

Rationales:
A. **Respiratory rate of 30 breaths/min**
The client is experiencing respiratory acidosis. Tachypnea does not produce compensation in respiratory acidosis.
B. **Apical rate of 120 beats/min**
Acid-base imbalances are compensated primarily by the lungs and the renal system. Plasma proteins and ionic shifts (intracellular) also serve as buffering systems. Tachycardia does not serve as a compensatory mechanism.
C. _Potassium level of 5.8 mmol/L (mEq/L)_
To compensate for the acidosis created by increased CO_2, K^+ ions are released from cellular proteins and H^+ ions take their place, bound to the proteins. The result is frequently serum hyperkalemia.
D. **Complaints of a pounding headache**
Headache may be a manifestation of CO_2 retention, but it is not a compensatory mechanism for respiratory acidosis.

10. **A client with chronic back pain is not receiving adequate pain relief from oral analgesics. Which alternative action should the nurse explore to promote the client's independence?**

Rationales:
A. **Ask the healthcare provider to increase the analgesic dosage.**
Although this intervention may improve pain relief, it may not promote self-care without increasing side effects that could affect the client's independence.
B. **Obtain a prescription for a second analgesic, to be given by the IV route.**
The IV route does not promote self-care and may cause additional side effects that interfere with the

client's ability to carry out activities of daily living independently.

C. *Consider the client's receptivity to complementary therapy.*

This action supports self-care without the high level of adverse effects associated with additional medication. It is the least invasive measure, and it promotes the active participation (self-care) of the client.

D. *Encourage counseling to prevent future addiction.*

Referrals may be needed, but the nurse should teach clients about potential problems with medications and measures to manage pain and maintain self-care.

Maternal-Newborn Nursing

11. A client at 41 weeks' gestation who is in active labor calls the nurse to report that her membranes have ruptured. The nurse performs a vaginal examination and discovers that the umbilical cord has prolapsed. Which intervention should the nurse implement first?

Rationales:

A. *Elevate the presenting fetal part off the cord.*

This action is the most critical intervention. The nurse must prevent compression of the cord by the presenting part because that would impair fetal circulation, leading to both morbidity and death.

B. *Cover the cord with sterile moist NS gauze.*

If the cord is protruding outside the vagina, this action should be taken to prevent drying of the Wharton's jelly. However, another nurse should do this while the first nurse maintains elevation of the presenting part off the cord.

C. *Prepare for an emergency cesarean delivery.*

This is implemented by the staff while the nurse keeps the presenting part elevated off the cord.

D. *Start O_2 by facemask at 10 L/min.*

Oxygen should be provided to the mother to increase oxygen delivery to the fetus via the placenta; however, another nurse should do this while first the nurse keeps the presenting part elevated off the cord.

12. A client at 39 weeks' gestation plans to have an epidural block when labor is established. What intervention(s) should the nurse be prepared to implement to prevent side effects? (Select all that apply.)

Rationales:

A. *Teach the client about the procedure and the effects of the epidural.*

Teaching is an important nursing intervention to alleviate anxiety, but it does not prevent hypotension, a side effect due to vasodilation caused by the epidural block.

B. *Place the client in a chair next to the bed.*

Epidural block reduces lower extremity sensation and movement to varying degrees. Any upright positions such as walking and standing may not be possible during epidural pain management and may not prevent side effects.

C. *Administer a bolus of 500 mL of normal saline solution.*

Prehydration increases maternal blood volume and prevents hypotension, which occurs as a result of vasodilation, a side effect of epidural anesthesia. A saline solution is used to prevent fetal secretion of insulin that later places the neonate at risk for hypoglycemia.

D. *Monitor the fetal heart rate and contractions continuously.*

Vital signs should be monitored every 5 minutes immediately after the initial epidural dose, and if the client's condition is stable, then every 15 minutes.

E. *Assist the client to empty her bladder every 2 hours.*

Assisting the client to void every 2 hours prevents bladder distention.

13. A female client presents in the emergency department with right lower quadrant abdominal pain and pain in her right shoulder. She has no vaginal bleeding, and her last menses was 6 weeks ago. Which action should the nurse take first?

Rationales:

A. *Assess for abdominal rebound pain, distention, and fever.*

Bleeding related to an ectopic pregnancy (based on the client's history) may present these manifestations, but the nurse should first assess the client for hypovolemic shock.

B. *Obtain vital signs and IV access, and notify the healthcare provider.*

The nurse should first evaluate the client for vital sign changes of shock due to a ruptured ectopic pregnancy (an obstetrical emergency). A vascular access is vital in an emergency situation, and the healthcare provider should be notified immediately.

C. *Observe for recent musculoskeletal injury, bruising, or abuse.*

This may be part of the assessment if a life-threatening situation is ruled out first.

D. *Collect specimens for pregnancy test, hemoglobin, and white blood cell count.*

Specimens for a pregnancy test and complete blood count should be collected. However, the nurse should first notify the healthcare provider of the client's status, based on the presenting vital signs and symptoms of bleeding, as manifested by intraabdominal bleeding that collects under the diaphragm, causing referred shoulder pain.

14. A nurse has been assigned a pregnant client who has heart disease. The client's condition has been diagnosed as New York Heart Association (NYHA) Class II cardiac disease. What important fact(s) about activities of daily living while

pregnant should the nurse teach this client? (Select all that apply.)

Rationales:

A. *Increase fiber in the diet.*
Restrictions in activities of daily living for clients with NYHA Class II cardiac disease create a risk factor for constipation.

B. *Anticipate the need for rest breaks after physical activity.*
Individuals with NYHA Class II cardiac disease may have limitations on activity.

C. *Notify the healthcare provider if her rings do not fit.*
Tight rings may indicate weight gain, and the client may be at risk for congestive heart failure.

D. *Maintain bed rest with bathroom privileges.*
It is not necessary to maintain bed rest for a client with NYHA Class II cardiac disease.

E. *Start a low-impact aerobic program.*
Individuals with NYHA Class II cardiac disease may have some slight limitation of activity. During pregnancy, women may progress from Class I or II to Class III or IV as cardiac output increases and more stress is placed on the heart.

Medical-Surgical: Renal

15. A client is returning to the unit after an intravenous pyelogram (IVP). Which intervention should the nurse include in the plan of care?

Rationales:

A. *Maintain bed rest.*
There is no need to restrict mobility after an IVP.

B. *Increase fluid intake.*
The client should increase the fluid intake to clear the dye used in an IVP because the dye may damage the kidneys.

C. *Monitor for hematuria.*
There is no risk of hematuria related to an IVP.

D. *Continue NPO (nothing by mouth) status.*
The client does not need to be NPO after an IVP. Fluids should be increased.

16. The nurse is teaching a client who has chronic urinary tract infections about a prescription for ciprofloxacin (Cipro) 500 mg PO bid (twice daily). What side effect(s) could the client expect while taking this medication? (Select all that apply.)

Rationales:

A. *Photosensitivity*
This is a side effect of Cipro; exposure to sunlight or tanning beds should be avoided. The client should be instructed to use sunscreen and protective clothing.

B. *Dyspepsia*
Cipro causes gastrointestinal irritation, nausea and vomiting, and abdominal pain, which should be reported.

C. *Diarrhea*
Watery, foul-smelling diarrhea is an adverse reaction to Cipro that indicates pseudomembranous colitis; this should be reported and requires immediate intervention.

D. *Urinary frequency*
Urinary frequency may indicate that the medication is ineffective and should be reported.

E. *Pernicious anemia*
This is not a side effect of Cipro.

17. Which client complaint of pain requires the nurse's immediate intervention?

Rationales:

A. *Bladder pain while receiving a continuous saline irrigant 2 hours after a transurethral prostatic resection*
This client is at risk of clot formation occluding the catheter, and the pain may indicate bleeding and bladder distention; the nurse should evaluate this client immediately.

B. *Incisional pain on postoperative day 3 after a nephrectomy; the client requests an as-needed (PRN) oral pain medication*
This is not as high a priority compared with option A because the client is not at risk of altered homeostasis.

C. *Flank pain that is partially relieved when the client passes a renal calculus*
This client's condition is not likely to worsen now that the stone was passed; it should be evaluated after the client in option A.

D. *Bladder spasms after draining 1000 mL of urine during insertion of an indwelling catheter*
This client's pain reflects the bladder spasms and is a lower priority than option A.

18. A male client with a peritoneal dialysis catheter calls to report he feels poorly and has a fever. What is the best response by the clinic nurse?

Rationales:

A. *Encourage him to come to the clinic today for assessment.*
PD catheters are used in peritoneal dialysis. They are often used at home by the client, placing the client at risk for peritoneal infection. Because dialysis clients usually have some degree of compromised immunity and anemia, the client should come to the clinic for assessment.

B. *Instruct him to increase his fluid intake to 3 L/day.*
Clients who need dialysis retain fluid and usually are restricted to an intake that is only 300 mL greater than output.

C. *Review his medication regimen for adherence.*
The nurse should evaluate the client's adherence, but assessing him for infection is a higher priority.

D. *Inquire about his recent dietary intake of protein and iron.*

Iron deficiency and protein loss are common problems in clients who are receiving peritoneal dialysis. Dietary intake is important, but it is not a higher priority than possible infection.

Medical-Surgical: Cardiovascular

19. **The nurse is reviewing the cardiac markers for a client who was admitted immediately after reporting chest pain. Which marker is the best to determine cardiac damage?**

Rationales:
A. *Troponin levels*
   A rise in the troponin levels is diagnostic of myocardial injury and is considered the gold standard.
B. *Myoglobin level*
   An increase in myoglobin is indicative of muscle damage but is not specific to cardiac damage.
C. *Creatine kinase-MB level*
   This isoenzyme is useful for supporting a diagnosis of myocardial infarction and in determining the extent and time of the infarct.
D. *Lactate dehydrogenase (LDH) level*
   The LDH level is not currently used to determine recent cardiac damage.

20. **The nurse is providing discharge instructions to a client who has been diagnosed with angina pectoris. Which instruction is most important?**

Rationales:
A. *Avoid activity that involves the Valsalva maneuver.*
   Although minimizing or avoiding the Valsalva maneuver decreases anginal pain; this is not the most important factor.
B. *Seek emergency treatment if chest pain persists after the third nitroglycerin dose.*
   This instruction is most important because chest pain characteristic of acute myocardial infarction persists longer than 15 minutes, and delaying medical treatment can be life threatening.
C. *Rest for 30 minutes after having chest pain before resuming activity.*
   Waiting 30 minutes may be recommended only if the nitroglycerin is effective in relieving the chest pain.
D. *Keep extra nitroglycerin in an airtight, light-resistant bottle.*
   This is excellent medication teaching, but it does not have the same urgency as seeking emergency care.

21. **The nurse is providing discharge teaching for a client who has been prescribed diltiazem. Which dietary instruction has the highest priority?**

Rationales:
A. *Maintain a low-sodium diet.*
   The client may need to restrict sodium intake, but it is not specific for diltiazem.

B. *Eat a banana each morning.*
   If the client has low potassium, this should be recommended.
C. *Ingest high-fiber foods daily.*
   This is an excellent teaching point for everyone, but it is not specific for diltiazem.
D. *Avoid grapefruit products.*
   Grapefruit should be avoided during therapy with calcium channel blockers because it can cause an increase in the serum drug level, predisposing the client to hypotension.

22. **The nurse is teaching a young adult female who has a history of Raynaud's disease how to control her pain. What information should the nurse offer?**

Rationales:
A. *Take oral analgesics at regularly spaced intervals.*
   Pain is not always associated with Raynaud's disease, as is the feeling of cold hands and fingers and pallor. If pain is sporadic or situational, it should not require regular use of analgesics.
B. *Avoid extremes of heat and cold.*
   In Raynaud's disease, vascular spasms of the hands and fingers are triggered by exposure to extremes of heat or cold, which causes the characteristic pallor and cold-to-the-touch symptoms of the upper extremities.
C. *Limit food and fluids that contain caffeine.*
   Caffeine is not the primary trigger of the episodes; however, if the client notes that caffeine contributes to the blanching and coldness, it should be avoided.
D. *Keep the affected extremities in a dependent position.*
   This is not effective for a client with Raynaud's disease.

23. **The nurse is caring for a client taking warfarin for atrial fibrillation. Which client need should the nurse give highest priority?**

Rationales:
A. *Having protamine sulfate available*
   Protamine sulfate is the antidote for heparin.
B. *Teaching the client the importance of walking 10,000 steps daily*
   Low-impact exercise, such as walking, is best for clients prescribed Coumadin; however, this is not the highest priority.
C. *Encouraging the client to eat Brussels sprouts and cabbage*
   Brussels sprouts and cabbage are foods high in vitamin K and would not be encouraged.
D. *Monitoring the platelet count for indications of thrombocytopenia*
   Thrombocytopenia is a low platelet count. Platelets are essential for initiating the normal clotting mechanism. Coumadin therapy puts this client at risk for injury and bleeding.

Medical-Surgical: Respiratory

24. A client who was admitted to the hospital with cancer of the larynx is scheduled for a laryngectomy tomorrow. What is the client's priority learning need tonight?

Rationales:
A. *Anticipated body image changes*
   This is a concern after surgery, when the immediate life-threatening insult of cancer has been assimilated and basic needs have been met.
B. *Pain management expectations*
   Pain relief expectations are a priority, but the inability to convey (communicate) a subjective symptom, such as pain, is the fear the client perceives first.
C. *Communication techniques*
   A client who is in crisis and anticipating the immediate postoperative period is concerned with immediate needs, such as the ability to express and convey a subjective symptom (e.g., pain) and obtain intervention.
D. *Postoperative nutritional needs*
   Nutrition is important to promote healing, but the ability to communicate subjective needs is a higher priority.

Psychiatric Nursing

25. A victim of a motor vehicle collision is dead on arrival at the emergency department. What action should the nurse implement to assist the spouse with this crisis?

Rationales:
A. *Ask whether there is family, friends, or clergy to call.*
   The nurse should help the spouse identify support systems and resources that are helpful in coping with a crisis situation, such as the sudden death of a spouse.
B. *Talk about the former relationship with the spouse.*
   The spouse may be unable to process information during the crisis, and the nurse should focus on immediate needs for coping and support.
C. *Provide education about the stages of grief and loss.*
   Educating the client about grief and loss is not an immediate priority in a crisis and should be provided after the spouse begins to cope with the situation.
D. *Assess the spouse's level of anxiety.*
   Although the nurse should assess the spouse for anxiety, the immediate intervention should include a directive approach to assist the spouse in dealing with the stressful event.

26. The nurse is planning to lead a seminar for community health nurses on violence against women during pregnancy. Which statement describes an appropriate technique for assessing for violence?

Rationales:
A. *Women should be assessed only if they are part of high-risk groups.*
   Violence against women occurs in all ethnic groups and at all income levels.
B. *Women may be assessed in the presence of young children but not intimate partners.*
   It is important to assess women without their partners present; it is also important that verbal children not be present because they may repeat what is heard. Infants may be present.
C. *Women should be assessed once during pregnancy.*
   Many women do not reveal violence the first time they are asked. As trust develops between the nurse and the client, the woman may be more comfortable sharing her story. Also, violence may start later in the pregnancy.
D. *Women should be reassessed face to face by a nurse as the pregnancy progresses.*
   More than one face-to-face interview elicits the highest reports of violence during pregnancy.

27. The charge nurse reminds clients on the mental health unit that breakfast is at 8 AM, medications are given at 9 AM, and group therapy sessions begin at 10 AM. Which treatment modality has been implemented?

Rationales:
A. *Milieu therapy*
   Milieu therapy uses resources and activities in the environment to assist with improving social functioning and activities of daily living.
B. *Behavior modification*
   Behavior modification involves changing behaviors using positive and negative reinforcements to allow desired activities or remove privileges.
C. *Peer therapy*
   Peer therapy is not a single therapeutic modality; it involves the interaction of peers who are responsible for supporting, sharing, and compromising within their peer group and milieu.
D. *Problem solving*
   Problem solving is used in crisis intervention; it focuses on problem identification and ways to return to previous levels of functioning.

28. The nurse is accompanying a male client to the radiography department when he becomes panic stricken at the elevator and states, "I can't get on that elevator." Which action should the nurse take first?

Rationales:
A. *Ask one more staff member to ride the elevator.*
   One more staff member will not be able to mobilize the client to ride the elevator, because he client must first recognize his feelings about the phobia and accept the need to change his behavior.

B. Offer a prescribed antianxiety medication.
Offering an antianxiety medication may be needed to proceed with desensitization.

C. Begin desensitization about riding the elevator.
Desensitizing the client may be implemented, but first the client should identify his fears and recognize his anxiety.

D. _Affirm the client's fears about riding the elevator._
The nurse should first validate and allow the client to affirm his anxiety and fears about riding the elevator. Then options to initiate desensitization may be considered.

29. **A male client who experiences frequent nightmares and somnambulism is found one night trying to strangle his roommate. Which intervention is the nurse's highest priority?**

Rationales:

A. Give the client a sedative or hypnotic.
Sleepwalking is more likely to occur when a client is fatigued and anxious and has received a hypnotic or sedative; safety is the priority.

B. Administer an antipsychotic medication.
An antipsychotic medication is indicated if the client is psychotic and agitated; however, the nurse should ensure the safety of both clients first.

C. _Assign a UAP to sit with the client._
The nurse should implement safety precautions immediately and place a sitter with the patient.

D. Process with both clients about the event.
Although both clients should talk about the incident, this is not an opportune time, and the clients should be separated to provide a safe environment.

30. **The nurse is updating the plan of care for a client who has a borderline personality disorder. Which intervention is most important to implement?**

Rationales:

A. _Always assign the same nurse to care for the client._
The best intervention is to provide consistency and avoid splitting by assigning the client to only one nurse.

B. Avoid challenging inappropriate behavior.
The nurse should assist the client to recognize manipulative behavior and set limits on manipulative behaviors as necessary.

C. Limit the client's contact with other clients.
Socialization should be encouraged to improve the client's social skills.

D. Remove consequences for acting-out behavior.
Firm limits with clear expectations and consequences are needed for manipulative clients.

31. **A female adolescent is admitted to the mental health unit for anorexia nervosa. In planning care, what is the nurse's priority intervention?**

Rationales:

A. Teach the client the importance of self-expression.
Self-expression of feelings is important, but reestablishing normal eating habits and physiological integrity is the priority intervention.

B. _Supervise the client's activities during the day._
The nurse should monitor and supervise the client's activities to prevent binging, purging, or avoiding meals.

C. Include the client in daily group therapy.
The client should be included in daily groups, but the priority is physiological needs and monitoring meals.

D. Facilitate social interactions with others.
The client should be given opportunities to socialize, but monitoring activities during the day, especially meals, is the priority.

32. **The charge nurse is planning the daily schedule for clients on the mental health unit. A male client who is manic should be assigned to which activity?**

Rationales:

A. A basketball game in the gym
The client should avoid any potentially competitive physical activity, especially contact sports, that can stimulate aggressive acting out.

B. _Jogging at least 1 mile_
Jogging is the best activity for this client because it is a noncompetitive physical activity, and it requires the use of large muscle groups that expend energy associated with mania.

C. A table tennis game with a peer
The client should not be assigned to any competitive activities that can frustrate him and stimulate mood swings.

D. Group therapy with the art therapist
A manic client may become disruptive and distracted in an art group; physical activity using large muscle groups is more effective in expending energy.

Leadership and Delegation

33. **A nurse is planning the client assignments for the night shift. The nursing team includes a registered nurse, a licensed practical nurse, and two unlicensed assistive personnel (UAP) on the nursing team. Which duties could be delegated to the UAPs? (Select all that apply.)**

Rationales:

A. _Transport a client who has had a stroke to the radiology department for a computed tomography (CT) scan._

B. Retrieve a unit of packed cells from the blood bank for a transfusion.

C. _Bathe a 25-year-old client with sickle cell disease who has multiple IV lines and a patient-controlled analgesia pump._

D. _Turn a 92-year-old client who has end-stage heart failure and a do-not-resuscitate order._

E. *Contact the healthcare provider for a client with a fingerstick blood glucose level of 49 mg/dL.*
The UAP can perform noninvasive and nonsterile activities (options A, C, and D); collect and report data such as vital signs, height and weight, and capillary blood glucose results; assist with socialization; and perform clerical duties (option E).

34. A hospitalized client has been newly diagnosed with type 2 diabetes. Which task(s) can the RN delegate to the UAP? (Select all that apply.)

Rationales:
A. *Contacting the dietitian for a prescribed consult*
B. *Reporting the client's insulin injection technique*
C. *Obtaining the fingerstick blood glucose level before each meal and at bedtime*
D. *Reminding the client to dry the toes carefully after a shower*
E. *Talking to the client about foods that raise the blood glucose level*
The UAP can collect and report data such as vital signs, height and weight, and capillary blood sugar results (option C); perform hygiene tasks (option D); and carry out clerical duties (option A). Clients who need education or reinforcement of education require intervention by the RN or PN (options B and E).

35. The home health nurse evaluates the insulin preparation and administration technique of a 36-year-old male client newly diagnosed with diabetes. The client has been prescribed insulin: lispro (Humalog) pen 10 units subcutaneously ac and Lantus 45 units subcutaneously once daily in the AM. Which finding indicates that the client needs further education?

Rationales:
A. *He mixes Lantus and lispro in the same syringe for the AM doses.*
Lantus must not be mixed with any other insulin or dilutions.
B. *He leaves the insulin syringe in place for 5 seconds after injection.*
The pen must be held with the needle in place for 5 seconds to ensure that all insulin has been injected.
C. *He stores the opened insulin vials at room temperature in the cabinet.*
Insulin is stored at room temperature, out of direct sunlight.
D. *He recaps and disposes of the single-use insulin syringe.*
Clients may recap needles, but healthcare providers may not to reduce the risk of needlestick injury.

36. At change of shift, the charge nurse assigns the UAP four clients. The RN should direct the UAP to take vital signs on which client first?

Rationales:
A. *The 89-year-old with chronic obstructive pulmonary disease who is resting quietly on 2 L of oxygen and who needs assistance with a bath*
This client is stable.
B. *The client who returned from endoscopy about 30 minutes ago and is requesting something to eat*
This client needs to have his vital signs taken to determine his stability after endoscopy; this is a priority.
C. *The client newly diagnosed with type 2 diabetes who had a fingerstick blood glucose level of 4.2 mmol/L (75 mg/dL) and who needs help with breakfast*
This client is stable.
D. *The newly admitted client with rheumatoid arthritis who needs to have hand splints reapplied to both hands*
This client is stable.

37. After change-of-shift report, the nurse reviews her assignments. Which client should the nurse assess first?

Rationales:
A. *The elderly client receiving palliative care for heart failure who complains of constipation and nervousness*
Constipation and nervousness are expected and common complications of palliative care.
B. *An adult client admitted for possible pneumonia with a heart rate of 110 and a respiratory rate of 24.*
Tachycardia and tachypnea are two of the criteria for systemic inflammatory response syndrome (SIRS), signs of early sepsis. This client needs to be seen first.
C. *The middle-aged client with end-stage renal failure whose urinary output has been 95 mL for the past 8 hours*
Oliguria or anuria is an expected outcome in end-stage renal failure.
D. *The client who is 2 days postoperative from a thoracotomy and who has chest tubes, is on oxygen at 3 L/min, and has a respiratory rate of 12 breaths/min*
This respiratory rate is within normal limits.

38. The nurse is reviewing the laboratory values of her assigned clients. Which client has an abnormal laboratory report that the nurse should communicate immediately to the healthcare provider?

Rationales:
A. *The client who is post splenectomy after a motor vehicle accident and has a hemoglobin of 109 mmol/L (10.9 g/dL)*
This laboratory value may require action, but it is not the priority.
B. *The client receiving warfarin (Coumadin) who has an international normalized ratio (INR) of 2.3*
This lab value may require action, but it is not the priority.

C. *The 38-year-old client who is 24 hours post thyroidectomy and has a total calcium level of 2.35 mmol/L (9.4 mg/dL)*
This lab value may require action, but it is not the priority.

D. <u>*The newly admitted client who has a blood urea nitrogen (BUN) of 10.7 mmol/L (30 mg/dL) and a creatinine of 97 mcmol/L (1.1 mg/dL)*</u>
The normal BUN-to-creatinine ratio is 10-20:1. A BUN that is disproportionally elevated raises suspicion of dehydration; the nurse should notify the healthcare provider immediately.

39. **The nurse receives change of shift report on her four acute care clients. Which action should the nurse take first?**

Rationales:

A. <u>*Contact the healthcare provider for a prescription for an antiemetic on a postoperative client who has been vomiting.*</u>
Postoperative nausea and vomiting (PONV) are among the most common reactions after surgery. PONV can stress and irritate abdominal and gastrointestinal wounds, increase intracranial pressure in patients who had head and neck surgery, elevate intraocular pressure in patients who had eye surgery, and increase the risk for aspiration. Obtaining a prescription for relieving PONV will decrease these risks.

B. *Notify a family member of a client's impending transfer to the intensive care unit for angina and ST-segment changes.*
This is a change in status and should be performed after managing the PONV.

C. *Inform the healthcare provider of a potassium level of 5.2 mmol/L (mEq/L) in the client with end-stage renal disease.*
This is an expected outcome of end-stage renal disease.

D. *Begin assessment rounds, starting with the palliative care client having a diagnosis of congestive failure.*
Assessing the client receiving palliative care is important; however, managing the client with PONV is the priority.

40. **The emergency department staff nurse is assigned four clients. Which client should the nurse assess first?**

Rationales:

A. *A preschooler with a barking cough, an O_2 saturation of 93% on room air, and occasional inspiratory stridor*
This is not a medical emergency but may require intervention.

B. *A 10-month-old with a tympanic temperature of 38.9 °C (102 °F) and green nasal drainage and who is pulling at her ears*

This is not a medical emergency but may require intervention.

C. *A crying 8-month-old with a harsh, paroxysmal cough; an audible expiratory wheeze; and mild retractions*
This is not a medical emergency but may require intervention.

D. <u>*A clingy 3-year-old who has a sore throat and drooling and whose tongue slightly protrudes from his mouth*</u>
Drooling, a history of sore throat, and a protruding tongue are classic manifestations of epiglottitis; this is a medical emergency.

41. **The outpatient clinic nurse is reviewing phone messages from last night. Which client should the nurse call back first?**

Rationales:

A. <u>*A woman at 30 weeks' gestation who has been diagnosed with mild preeclampsia; she was unable to relieve her heartburn.*</u>
A sign of a potential complication of eclampsia is epigastric pain, which may be indicative of liver damage and HELLP (hemolysis, elevated liver enzymes, low platelet count) syndrome, a medical emergency.

B. *A woman at 24 weeks' gestation who was crying about painful vulvar lesions and urinary frequency for the past 8 hours*
This is a reasonable concern, but it does not take priority over option A.

C. *A woman at 12 weeks' gestation who was recently discharged from the hospital with hyperemesis gravidarum; she had had two episodes of vomiting in 6 hours*
This is a reasonable concern, but it does not take priority over option A.

D. *A woman with type 1 diabetes who tested positive with a home pregnancy kit; she was worried about managing her diabetes*
This is a reasonable concern, but it does not take priority over option A.

42. **The clinic nurse suspects that a 2-year-old child is being abused. Which assessment finding(s) would support this? (Select all that apply.)**

Rationales:

A. *Petechiae in a straight line on the chest*
Petechiae on the chest may be the result of the coining procedure, a cultural practice among Southeast Asian populations.

B. *Gray-blue pigmented areas on the sacral region*
These are Mongolian spots, blue areas commonly located on the sacral region that are consistent in shape and color.

C. <u>*Bald patches on the scalp*</u>
Bald patches typically are symmetrical and are indicative of physical abuse.

D. **Ear tugging and crying**
Ear tugging and crying are typical signs of otitis media.

E. **_Symmetrical burns on the hands_**
Symmetrical burns are indicative of physical abuse.

43. **The nurse is caring for a client who had a thoracotomy 48 hours ago and now has left lower lobe chest tubes. The nurse notes that a chest tube is not tidaling. Which action should the nurse take first?**

Rationales:

A. **_Check for kinks in the chest drainage system._**
Normal fluctuation of the water, called tidaling, reflects the intrapleural pressure during inspiration and expiration. If no tidaling is observed (rising with inspiration and falling with expiration in a spontaneously breathing patient), the drainage system may be blocked. An absence of fluctuation may mean that the lung has fully reexpanded or can mean that there is an obstruction in the chest tube. A simple step is to ensure that there are no kinks that would occlude the chest tube and prevent lung drainage and expansion.

B. **Assess the heart rate and blood pressure.**
Checking the heart rate and blood pressure is not directly related to the lack of chest tube drainage.

C. **Notify the rapid response team immediately.**
Although the nurse should immediately notify the rapid response team for tracheal deviation, sudden onset of dyspnea, or mediastinal shift, the absence of tidaling may not be a medical emergency.

D. **Momentarily disconnect from wall suction.**
Disconnecting the chest tube from wall suction will not affect tidaling or the water seal.

44. **While the nurse is caring for a client who has had a myocardial infarction, the monitor alarm sounds, and the nurse notes ventricular fibrillation. What is the nurse's first course of action?**

Rationales:

A. **Notify the healthcare provider.**
This may be an appropriate action after assessment of the client's clinical status.

B. **Increase the oxygen concentration.**
This may be an appropriate action after assessment of the client's clinical status.

C. **_Assess the client's level of consciousness._**
If a monitor alarm sounds, the nurse should first assess the client's clinical status to see whether the problem is an actual dysrhythmia or a monitoring system malfunction.

D. **Prepare to defibrillate the client.**
This may be an appropriate action after assessment of the client's clinical status.

45. **The healthcare provider has prescribed the removal of a client's internal jugular central line** catheter. To remove the catheter safely, the nurse should give which intervention(s) the highest priority? (Select all that apply.)

Rationales:

A. **Carefully remove the Bioderm dressing.**
Removing the Bioderm dressing is important, but it is not a safety priority.

B. **_Place the client in the Trendelenburg position._**
The procedure for removing the catheter safely is (1) place the client in the Trendelenburg position; (2) have the client take a deep breath and hold it; and (3) gently withdraw the catheter while applying direct pressure with sterile gauze. Holding the breath creates positive pressure in the intrathoracic space, and the Trendelenburg position minimizes the risk of air entering the catheter.

C. **Send the catheter tip to the lab for culture and sensitivity.**
The catheter tip may or may not be sent to the lab, depending on the protocol of the facility.

D. **_Have the client take a deep breath during removal._**

E. **Apply pressure for 20 minutes after removal of the catheter.**
Applying pressure for 20 minutes is a technique used in arterial line withdrawal to prevent bleeding.

46. **The nurse who usually works on the orthopedic surgery unit is floating to a cardiovascular unit. Which client would be best to assign to the float nurse?**

Rationales:

A. **Client scheduled for a heart catheterization this morning**
Preparing the client for a cardiac catheterization requires specialized information and would be best to assign to the nurse who usually works on the cardiovascular unit.

B. **Client admitted last night for chest pain.**
This client requires close monitoring by the nurse who has additional education about cardiac issues.

C. **_Client who underwent popliteal bypass surgery yesterday_**
This would require similar care to a client who had just had lower extremity orthopedic surgery and would be the safest assignment for this nurse.

D. **Client who has heart failure and is scheduled for a stress test today.**
Preparing the client for a stress test requires specialized information and would be best to assign to the nurse who usually works on the cardiovascular unit.

47. **The nurse is admitting a client who is a paraplegic and has a nonhealing pressure ulcer with a possible methicillin-resistant _Staphylococcus aureus_ infection. A UAP and PN are assigned to the RN's**

team. Which tasks should be delegated to the PN? (Select all that apply.)

Rationales:
A. *Place the client in isolation.*
   This task can be safely assigned to the UAP.
B. *Complete a dressing change.*
   This task is within the scope of practice for the PN.
C. *Assess and document the wound.*
   Initial assessment of a wound should be completed by the registered nurse.
D. *Insert a urinary catheter.*
   This task is within the scope of practice for the PN.
E. *Administer oral pain medications.*
   This task is within the scope of practice for the PN.

48. **The nursing supervisor calls the nurse on a step-down unit about the need to open up a bed for a transfer of an unstable patient from the medical unit. Which client should the nurse transfer to the medical unit in order to receive this unstable client?**

Rationales:
A. *A client admitted for an ST-elevation myocardial infarction (STEMI) who just returned from having a cardiac catheterization performed*
   This patient needs close monitoring for the first 24 hours and should remain on the step-down unit.
B. *A client diagnosed with congestive heart failure who is receiving furosemide IV twice a day*
   This patient could be safely taken care of on a medical-surgical unit.
C. *A client with possible Guillain-Barré syndrome who may need an exchange transfusion*
   This patient needs close monitoring and should remain in the step-down unit.
D. *A client in hypertensive crisis who is on a sodium nitroprusside drip.*
   Patients on a nitroprusside drip need frequent vital signs and close monitoring. This patient should remain on the step-down unit.

49. **When accessing the Pyxis, the nurse finds chlorpropamide in the drawer instead of the expected chlorpromazine. Which actions should the nurse take? (Select all that apply.)**

Rationales:
A. *Remove the tablets of chlorpropamide.*
B. *Notify the pharmacy about the mistake.*
C. *Place an incident occurrence report.*
D. *Be extra vigilant because the pharmacy is making mistakes.*
E. *Place a warning note on the Pyxis machine.*
   The nurse needs to ensure that others do not give the wrong medication, so the tablets of chlorpropamide need to be removed and returned to the pharmacy (option A). The pharmacy needs to be made aware of

the error (option B) and an incident report completed (option C) to help prevent the error in the future.

50. **The nurse is calling the healthcare provider (HCP) about a client's current needs. What is the best way to communicate?**

Rationales:
A. *Call the HCP with the request and a recommendation.*
   Letting the physician know the needs of the patient is important, but key information may be missed using this way to communicate.
B. *Use the SBAR (situation, background, assessment, recommendation) tool regardless of the means of communication.*
   Using the SBAR format ensures that all key information is given and is the best way to communicate.
C. *Send a text message or page with the needed order.*
   This may be an ineffective way to communicate and may not ensure that all key information is given..
D. *Ask the HCP to come back to the unit to discuss the client's needs.*
   Although face-to-face communication is often valuable, this does not ensure that all key information is communicated.

51. **The healthcare provider plans to do a paracentesis on a client with cirrhosis in 1 hour. In what order should the nurse perform the following activities?**

Rationales:
A. *Ensure that the informed consent has been obtained.*
B. *Measure the client's abdominal girth.*
C. *Have the patient empty his or her bladder.*
D. *Assemble needed equipment.*
E. *Administer oral pain medication.*

Rationales:
   Correct order: A, B, E, D, C.
   Before a procedure can be completed, it is essential to have an informed consent (A). Oral pain medication can then be given (after the consent has been obtained) to help the patient relax during the procedure but give the medication time to act (B). The client then needs to empty his or her bladder before the procedure to prevent accidentally puncturing the bladder (E). After the bladder is empty, a baseline abdominal girth is obtained (D). Finally, the nurse needs to assemble the correct equipment for the procedure (C).

52. **The nurse receives report on a client from the emergency department with a diagnosis of pneumonia. Which intervention has the highest priority?**

Rationales:

A. Obtain blood cultures.
Blood cultures are not needed unless the client is suspected of being septic.

B. _Initiate prescribed antibiotics._
Studies have shown that the sooner antibiotics are started, the better the outcomes. Current requirements include antibiotic administration within 2 hours of diagnosis. This is the priority.

C. Place the client in isolation.
The question does not state what organism is causing the pneumonia, so this is not essential.

D. Obtain an accurate weight.
This would be needed if the antibiotic is weight based but is not usually a priority.

---

53. The nurse is part of the triage team at a disaster. Which client should be seen first?

Rationales:

A. A 90-year-old woman with a crushed pelvis and head injuries
This client would be triaged black.

B. A 21-year-old male screaming in pain from a broken leg
This client's injuries are not life threatening, and he can wait to be seen.

C. _A 30-year-old woman with a flail chest secondary to a puncture wound_
The flail chest causes the heart to become unstable and is life threatening. This client needs to be seen immediately.

D. A 12-year-old crying with multiple small lacerations
Although the child needs to be comforted, the injuries are not life threatening, and this client can wait for treatment.

---

54. The triage nurse in the emergency room is assessing four (4) clients. Which client requires the most immediate intervention?

A. The adult client who arrived via ambulance with numbness and tingling of his left arm and face

B. The adult client who had a seizure at home who is sleeping on his left side

C. The 60-year-old client who complains of frequent urination and has a blood sugar of 16.7 mmol/L (300 mg/dL)

D. The middle-aged client who presents with severe unilateral back pain and previous history of kidney stones

Rationales:

A. _The client who arrived via ambulance with numbness and tingling of his left arm and face_
The client may be diagnosed with a brain attack and requires immediate assessment and interventions. If interventions are initiated quickly the complications may be mitigated.

B. The adult client who had a seizure at home who is sleeping on his left side
While a seizure is highly concerning, the priority is the client who may be diagnosed with a brain attack.

C. The 60-year-old client who complains of frequent urination and has a blood sugar of 16.7 mmol/L (300 mg/dL)
An elevated blood sugar may indicate diabetes. It is considered urgent and not emergent.

D. D. The middle-aged client who presents with severe unilateral back pain and previous history of kidney stones
Although this is highly concerning, the client who may have a stroke requires immediate attention.

---

55. After the change-of-shift report on an orthopedic floor, which client should the nurse assess first?

Rationales:

A. A client who had surgery yesterday and has a temperature of 37.6 °C (99.7 °F)
A slight increase in temperature is expected postoperatively.

B. _A client who is complaining of numbness and tingling distal to the fracture site_
This is a sign of compartment syndrome. This client needs to be assessed first.

C. A client who had a left leg amputation and states he is experiencing pain in the left foot.
Phantom pain is expected after an amputation and should be treated but is not as critical as assessing for compartment syndrome.

D. A client who is extremely upset with the care and is requesting to speak with the manager
This is a customer service issue and needs to be addressed but is not a high priority.

---

56. The nurse is administering medications to a client admitted for an overdose and a history of substance abuse. Which intervention(s) are priorities to include in this client's plan of care? (Select all that apply.)

Rationales:

A. Allow the client to take medications independently.
With a history of substance abuse, the nurse needs to observe the client as medications are taken.

B. _Ensure that all medications have been swallowed before leaving the client's room._
To ensure that medications are not being hoarded or kept to be taken at a later time, the nurse needs to watch the client swallow his or her medications.

C. _Request that oral pain medications be changed from tablet to oral suspension._
Liquid forms of medications are harder to save to be taken later so are often used for clients with a history of substance abuse.

D. Give Romazicon every 6 hours around the clock.
Romazicon is used to reverse benzodiazepine overdose and is given as needed, not around the clock.

E. Only give medications to the client via the intravenous route.

There is no indication to give medications intravenously.

57. **The nurse is returning phone calls to clients who are cared for at an outpatient mental health center. Which client should the nurse call first?**

Rationales:

A. **The young mother diagnosed with schizophrenia who is hearing voices say that they are pursuing her children**

This client is at risk for hurting herself or her children. She needs to be seen first.

B. **The elderly male at an assisted living facility who says he wants to end it all**

This client is at risk for committing suicide, but he lives in a facility where there is staff that the nurse can notify about his thoughts. The staff can stay with him until he can be brought into the clinic.

C. **The female client diagnosed with bipolar disorder who is manic and has not slept for 48 hours**

Although this client needs to be seen to have her medications adjusted, she is not the priority client.

D. **The teenager diagnosed with bulimia whose mother called and reported that she found her daughter purging**

This client does need to be seen but is not in imminent danger of hurting herself.

58. **An 18-year-old female is being discharged after delivering a healthy baby. She has a cousin whose baby died from sudden infant death syndrome (SIDS). The client seems to know many of the precautions to take. Which information does the nurse need to correct?**

Rationales:

A. **Always place infants on their backs to sleep.**

This is correct. Babies should be placed on their backs.

B. **Room sharing has been shown to decrease SIDS.**

This is correct. Studies show that room sharing does decrease SIDS.

C. **Keep the crib free of stuffed animals and crib pads.**

This is correct. The bed should be free of items that could cause suffocation.

D. **Sleeping with the baby can alert the mother to changes.**

Sleeping with the baby increases the risk for injury and SIDS for infants.

59. **A 4-year-old admitted with pneumonia weighs 18 kg. The healthcare provided has prescribed vancomycin 40 mg/kg/day IV. The order states to divide the dose and give it three times daily. How many mg of vancomycin should the child receive in each dose? (Round the answer to the nearest whole number.)**

_____ mg/dose

Rationales:

18 mg × 40 mg/kg = 720 mg/kg
720 mg / 3 = 240 mg/dose

60. **The nurse needs to initiate an IV on an 8-year-old child. Which intervention is appropriate?**

Rationales:

A. **Start the IV in the treatment room, not the child's room.**

The child's room is a safe zone, and painful treatments should not be performed in the child's room.

B. **Apply a lidocaine-based cream for a few minutes before starting the IV.**

To be effective, the cream needs to be applied for about 1 hour before the IV is started.

C. **Ask the parents to leave the room while performing the procedure.**

Having parents present can help the child cope with this procedure.

D. **Encourage the child to use guided imagery to cope.**

Children at this age are too young to understand and participate in guided imagery.